Percutaneous Breast Biopsy

Percutaneous Breast Biopsy

Editors

Steve H. Parker, M.D.
William E. Jobe, M.D.

Radiology Imaging Associates
Breast Diagnostic and Counseling Centre
Englewood, Colorado

Raven Press ⬧ New York

Raven Press, Ltd., 1185 Avenue of the Americas, New York, New York 10036

Made in the United States of America

Library of Congress Cataloging-in-Publication Data

Percutaneous breast biopsy / editors, Steve H. Parker, William E. Jobe.
     p. cm.
    Includes bibliographical references and index.
    ISBN 0-7817-0010-8
    1. Breast—Biopsy, Needle.   2. Breast—Cancer—Diagnosis.
  I. Parker, Steve H.   II. Jobe, William E.
    [DNLM: 1. Breast Diseases—diagnosis.   2. Biopsy—methods.
  3. Ultrasonography, Mammary.   WP 815 P429 1993]
  RC280.B8P38 1993
  616.99'449075—dc20
  DNLM/DLC   93-14055
  for Library of Congress   CIP

9 8 7 6 5 4 3 2 1

To our wives, Maggie and Sally, who have not only put up with the writing of this book, but also our inherent mischievous personalities.

Contents

Contributing Authors

Joan P. Camp, R.N.   *Radiology Imaging Associates, Breast Diagnostic and Counseling Centre, 8200 East Belleview Avenue #102, Englewood, Colorado 80111*

Mark A. Dennis, M.D.   *Radiology Imaging Associates, Breast Diagnostic and Counseling Centre, 8200 East Belleview Avenue #124, Englewood, Colorado 80111*

Laurie L. Fajardo, M.D.   *Department of Radiology, University of Arizona Health Sciences Center, 1501 North Campbell Avenue #1535, Tucson, Arizona 85724*

R. Edward Hendrick, Ph.D.   *Department of Radiology, University of Colorado Health Sciences Center, Campus Box C278, 4200 East Ninth Avenue, Denver, Colorado 80262*

William E. Jobe, M.D.   *Radiology Imaging Associates, Breast Diagnostic and Counseling Centre, 8200 East Belleview Avenue #124, Englewood, Colorado 80111*

Steve H. Parker, M.D.   *Radiology Imaging Associates, Breast Diagnostic and Counseling Centre, 8200 East Belleview Avenue #124, Englewood, Colorado 80111*

Peter J. Philpott, M.D.   *Department of Pathology, Swedish Medical Center, 501 East Hampden Avenue, Englewood, Colorado 80110*

Gina Simon, R.T.R.   *Radiology Imaging Associates, Breast Diagnostic and Counseling Centre, 8200 East Belleview Avenue #102, Englewood, Colorado 80111*

A. Thomas Stavros, M.D.   *Radiology Imaging Associates, Breast Diagnostic and Counseling Centre, 8200 East Belleview Avenue #124, Englewood, Colorado 80111*

John E. Truell, M.D.   *Department of Pathology, Swedish Medical Center, 501 East Hampden Avenue, Englewood, Colorado 80110*

Foreword

There is overwhelming evidence that the sooner breast carcinoma is diagnosed, the better the outcome. Scientific proof that early detection of breast cancer through mammographic screening significantly decreases mortality from the disease can be considered one of the major accomplishments of the radiology profession. This achievement has not come about through merely interpreting standard mammograms.

Although screening is based upon the interpretation of two-view mammograms, the diagnosis of breast diseases requires not only a thorough mammographic workup, but also an intelligent use of adjunctive methods. Our ultimate goal is to provide as accurate a preoperative diagnosis as possible, preferably including microscopic diagnosis. It should be remembered that the success of the population-based mammography screening programs was in part due to the use of fine-needle aspiration biopsy. Cytologic diagnosis enabled a team to efficiently restrict surgical biopsies. Further development of large-core needle biopsy technique, combined with stereotactic instrumentation, has considerably strengthened the armamentarium of the radiologist.

This book provides comprehensive coverage of the most useful adjunctive method presently available: large-core needle biopsy. The authors have played a decisive role in the development and acceptance of this technique. Importantly, the role of fine-needle aspiration biopsy is also carefully evaluated.

This pioneer work is remarkable in that the authors have foreseen the impact of large-core needle biopsy upon breast diagnosis and have succeeded in refining the professional environment necessary for its successful application.

The emphasis is on teamwork. The new role of the radiologist includes directing the individual diagnostic and interventional procedures, and in a broader sense, taking responsibility for coordinating the preoperative diagnostic workup. This places the radiologist in the role of the quarterback.

Close cooperation with the surgeon, pathologist, and oncologist (as outlined in this book) is mandatory for the success of modern diagnosis and treatment of breast diseases. This book is indeed a timely publication.

Laszlo Tabar, M.D.

Preface

Radiologists are diagnosticians. In the breast, however, their role has been hampered by the lack of specificity in imaging techniques and by radiologic and surgical dogma that is out-of-date and no longer appropriate. At Radiology Imaging Associates' Breast Diagnostic and Counseling Centre, we have developed a new approach to diagnosing breast lesions. We believe that this approach offers dramatic advantages over existing protocols and techniques. Therefore, this book is intended not only as a primer on the technique of percutaneous breast biopsy, but as a resource for those who are looking for a more logical approach to the definitive diagnosis of breast lesions.

All of the chapters in this book are integral pieces in the breast diagnosis puzzle. Readers are encouraged to first read Chapters 7 (*Stereotactic Large-Core Breast Biopsy*) and 13 (*Ultrasound-Guided Large-Core Breast Biopsy*) to familiarize themselves with the basic techniques of percutaneous breast biopsy. This should help clarify the material in other chapters, which flesh out details of the technique from different perspectives.

The first section of this book is a general overview, which includes a brief history of the mammographic, ultrasonographic, and interventional techniques that led to the development of percutaneous breast biopsy. There is a chapter on needle selection, and chapters discussing percutaneous breast biopsy from the pathologist's, nurse's, and technologist's perspectives.

The second section covers stereotactic breast biopsy, including a physicist's description of principles of stereotactic mammography and quality assurance. Although we strongly believe that stereotactic breast biopsy should be performed using the recumbent, automated, large-core technique described in Chapter 7, for completeness we have included chapters on breast fine-needle aspiration biopsy and add-on stereotactic units, graciously contributed by Laurie Fajardo. We have added editors' notes at the end of each of these two chapters detailing our position.

The third section deals with ultrasound applications in the breast. Unfortunately, breast ultrasound has been so poorly portrayed in the existing literature that it is underutilized by most radiologists. However, the tools described in the four chapters on breast ultrasound are essential to the diagnostic armamentarium of modern breast radiologists. The first three chapters of that section are crucial preparation for the final chapter on ultrasound-guided breast biopsy.

A final chapter touches on the future of percutaneous breast biopsy. New developments such as the charged coupled device for obtaining digitized stereotactic images are mentioned, and some as yet undiscovered possibilities are suggested.

The scope of this book extends beyond percutaneous breast biopsy to include a global approach to breast imaging. We believe this makes it a much more valuable resource to radiologists interested in the diagnosis of breast disease. We firmly believe that the tools offered herein will enable radiologists to meet the needs of 21st century women who will demand, and rightfully so, that the old 19th and 20th century diagnostic methods be discarded. With the protocols and techniques described in this book, the radiologist's role in the *definitive* diagnosis of breast disease is just beginning.

Steve H. Parker, M.D.
William E. Jobe, M.D.

Acknowledgment

We are deeply grateful to Lisa Hofsess for her indispensible assistance in preparing this book. In light of the exigencies of private practice radiology, this book would have been impossible without her help. We will always be indebted to her.

Percutaneous Breast Biopsy, edited by
Steve H. Parker and William E. Jobe.
Raven Press, Ltd., New York © 1993.

CHAPTER 1

Historical Perspectives

William E. Jobe

BEFORE IMAGING

Percutaneous breast biopsy ushers in a new era in the battle against breast cancer. However, this is only another incremental step in a fight that began long ago.

In the mid-nineteenth century, treatment for breast cancer, removal of the entire breast, was predominantly palliative (i.e., intended to prevent the cancer from invading the skin and creating an open wound). Usually, treatment was sought and/or given only after a breast mass had reached what would be considered enormous proportions by today's standards. In 1853, Dr. James Paget wrote about breast cancer that "we have never observed the failure of recurrence over a seven year period. Our decision in individual cases for or against removal of a carcinomatous breast was never based on hope of curing the disease" (1). In 1856, Dr. A. Velpeau, a French surgeon, observed that "the disease always recurs after surgery. In fact the course of disease is accelerated by surgery and the fatal end occurs sooner" (1). Then Dr. D. H. Agnew stated, in 1883, "I do not doubt that cancer will one day be curable but I do not believe that this will be procured through the surgeon's scalpel" (1).

In 1894, Dr. William Halstead (2) published his first paper on a new surgical treatment for breast carcinoma—removal *en bloc* of the tumor, its adjacent muscle and other tissue structures, and the draining lymph system. Dr. Halstead noted in his article that few patients had survived breast cancer longer than three years. He measured his surgical success in terms of four-year survival.

In 1905, Dr. Steinthal further defined surgical indications and promoted the dictum that every palpable nodule must be removed surgically and examined histologically (1). A short time later, Dr. Haagensen applied vast amounts of experimental data to the improvement of surgical and palpation techniques. More importantly, his data led to refinements in prognosis and thus to better indications of inoperability (3).

BREAST RADIOLOGY

Unfortunately, the only approach to diagnosis in the nineteenth century was palpation and, as noted above, lesions were not detected or treated until they were very large. Given that better surgical treatment was becoming available, earlier diagnosis of much smaller lesions was necessary. In 1895, Dr. Wilhelm Konrad Roentgen (a physicist) discovered the x-ray and the field of radiologic imaging was born. The technology was dispersed literally within weeks of its discovery.

All of the early work with breast imaging was led by surgeons. In 1913, Dr. A. Salomon (4), at the University of Berlin, was the first to use x-ray to look at breast tissue. He studied surgical specimens after mastectomy, recording roentgenologic signs of cancer characteristics, including calcifications. It was not until the late 1920s that the field of mammography emerged and the breast was imaged *in vivo*. Dr. Otto Kleinschmidt (5), a German surgeon, published the first image of the breast in Dr. Payr's textbook of surgery.

Dr. Payr's work in breast imaging spanned over 30 years. Radiologists eventually became interested, led by the South Americans Dominguez and Goyanes; the Americans, Warren, Reis, and Seabold; and Vogel in Germany. In the late 1930s, Dr. Jacob Gershon-Cohen and Dr. Albert Strickler pioneered work imaging the normal breast. Raoul Leborgne (6), a student of Dominguez, defined the importance of calcifications, differ-

W.E. Jobe: Radiology Imaging Associates, Breast Diagnostic and Counseling Centre, Englewood, Colorado 80111.

entiating among malignant and benign calcifications and those associated with fibroadenomas.

There was a temporary hiatus until Dr. Robert Egan developed a standardized mammography technique in the late 1950s. He also began to define imaging patterns of breast carcinoma. More importantly, however, he created the "team-teaching concept." Through the American College of Radiology, he devised a teaching method to reach local community hospitals across the United States. This first interdisciplinary teaching approach on a national level was a milestone in medical education (7).

In 1966, Dr. John Wolfe (8) in Detroit refined the Xerox process of breast imaging and diagnosis that had been developed by John Roach and Herman Hilleboe. The Xerox process improved the resolution of breast imaging and added further diagnostic criteria, including subtle signs of cancer, parenchymal patterns, and linear tumor growth. Edge enhancement allowed margin pattern recognition to become more important.

CORRELATING RADIOLOGY WITH PATHOLOGY

Dr. John Martin in Houston, Texas, organized one of the first formal collaborations between a radiologist and a pathologist. Dr. Martin, a radiologist, and Dr. Steve Gallagher, a pathologist, correlated whole-organ mounts of breast tumor with radiographic images. Their work further improved pattern recognition of cancer within the breast and introduced the concept of minimal breast cancer (9,10).

In a review article in the first edition of *Radiologic Clinics of North America,* Gershon-Cohen and Berger (11) presented a conceptual approach to mammography which correlated imaging and pathologic structures to define tumor growth. In 1960 Dr. Gershon-Cohen and Dr. Helen Ingleby, a pathologist with an abiding interest in the breast, wrote the classic treatise, *Comparative Anatomy, Pathology, and Roentgenology of the Breast* (12). Although now out of print, this volume remains an indispensable addition to the library of every radiologist interested in breast imaging.

THE CONTRIBUTION OF INDUSTRY

The contribution of the industrial manufacturers should also be recognized. The French company, Compagnie Generale de Radiologie (CGR), designed the first dedicated mammography unit at the direction of the French radiologist, Dr. Charles Gros. Other units soon followed. Dedicated mammography equipment and the recognition of the importance of breast imaging soon led to the formation of a breast subdivision within radiologic departments across the country.

At the same time, radiologists were urging film companies to recognize the potential market for dedicated film. Dupont and Kodak were leaders in this area and were key to improving resolution and diagnostic capability. John Fink of Kodak, Robert Wayrynen of Dupont, and Bill Loranger of Xerox prodded their own hierarchies into realizing the importance of breast imaging. Their clear insight into the problem of breast cancer facilitated the film industry's understanding of its important contribution.

DOSE REDUCTION

In conjunction with the manufacturing groups, radiologic physicists and radiologists with a deep understanding of physics contributed to the development of better breast imaging. Perhaps more importantly, they pioneered reductions in radiation dose. Radiation dose reduction was influenced tremendously by a critique of the cost-benefit ratio of radiation exposure by Dr. John Bailer (13) published in 1976 in the *Annals of Internal Medicine.* This article, picked up by the media, stimulated research that led to a marked decrease in exposure dose to patients. Despite the positive outcome of this incident, the sad experience with a radiation scare overplayed by the media should not be ignored. Better communication and a decrease in radiologists' own arrogance could have prevented it.

Nor should the ability of the media to reach and positively influence the public be overlooked. The successful treatment of breast cancer diagnosed early in several presidents' wives and other publicly notable women has increased public awareness of breast cancer and the importance of mammographic screening.

ORGANIZATIONAL CONTRIBUTIONS

The contributions of medical organizations, especially the American College of Radiology (ACR), the American Medical Association, the American College of Surgeons, the American College of Pathology, and the American College of Obstetrics and Gynecology should be applauded. These organizations publicly supported screening mammography for early detection of breast cancer. Their credibility helped encourage women to get mammograms before lesions grew to a palpable size.

The American College of Radiology committee on breast disease, chaired by Dr. Wendell Scott, staffed by Bill Melton and Dr. Bob Harrington, and encouraged by Bill Stronach, Executive Director of the American College of Radiology, introduced a new concept—interdisciplinary education of physicians. A team of radiologists, surgeons, and pathologists first educated community radiologists in mammography and then educated their surgical and pathologic colleagues in a team approach to the diagnosis and treatment of early breast disease.

Soon the radiotherapists started teaming up with the surgeons to offer women more conservative breast therapy. Led by such pioneers as Dr. Gilbert Fletcher and Dr. Eleanor Montague at Houston and Dr. J. R. Harris and Dr. Sam Hellman and their surgical colleague, Dr. Simon, at Boston, these teams helped reverse the perception of the inevitable fatality of breast cancer. Combining radiotherapy with new tissue preservation techniques produced better postsurgical cosmesis and was shown to cure breast cancer in many cases.

The American Cancer Society (ACS), the United States Department of Public Health through the Cancer Control Program, and the National Cancer Institute (NCI) also helped change public perception of breast disease. Mammography projects funded by these organizations led to today's concept of screening the entire U.S. population with mammography to improve early diagnosis of breast cancer. Dr. Philip Strax directed a mammography and palpation screening program sponsored by the health insurance plan of New York (HIP) from 1963 to 1966 (14). Heeding the advice of the ACR, the ACS and the NCI created the Breast Cancer Detection Demonstration Project (BCDDP) and other similar programs, which remain in effect in the United States today.

The success of these projects stimulated progress in other countries as well. The best known experience is that of Dr. Laszlo Tabar, a radiologist from Falun, Sweden, who is now sharing his findings with his radiologic colleagues around the world. The results of Tabar and Fagerberg's "two-county" screening program confirmed that screening mammography can significantly reduce breast cancer mortality (15). In addition to Dr. Tabar's landmark research efforts, his dedication to teaching has single-handedly brought the international radiologic community an organized, systematic approach to the radiologic workup of suspected breast lesions.

HOOK WIRES AND STEREOTACTIC MAMMOGRAPHY

During the late 1960s and early 1970s, developments in the fight against breast cancer focused on refining the diagnostic biopsy of nonpalpable lesions. Because the vast majority of these biopsies were blind surgical procedures, accurate prebiopsy localization needed to be developed. In 1963 Dr. Gerry Dodd performed what was probably the first needle localization (16). Prebiopsy localization using standard needles was rapidly replaced with techniques using special hook wires for better fixation (see Chapter 2).

Needle and hook wire placement became more accurate with stereotactic mammography. Stereotactic mammography was introduced first in Sweden in 1976 (17) and then in the United States in the mid-1980s by Dr. Kambiz Dowlatshahi. The first widely used stereotactic mammography units were attached to existing mammography equipment, and the localization or biopsy was performed with the patient sitting upright. As it became apparent that motion problems and patient comfort could not be adequately addressed with these units, dedicated recumbent units began to take hold. Currently, stereotactic units can target lesions within ± 1 mm.

Stereotactic breast biopsies with dedicated and with "add-on" units are discussed in Chapters 7 and 8, respectively.

BREAST ULTRASOUND

In 1947, Dr. Doug Howery and his coworkers constructed the first B-mode scanner in his basement, first using a tub and then a stock water tank as the water bath. Later, Howery and Dr. Joseph Holmes obtained the first ultrasound images of the human body in the basement of the radiology department of the University of Colorado Medical Center. They immersed patients in an old World War II B-29 bomber gun turret filled with water. Sound waves were then sent through the water bath, and the first ultrasound images of the liver were obtained (Joe Holmes, *personal communication*, 1960).

A short time later, the first breast ultrasound examinations were performed by Dr. Wild in 1951, Dr. Wagai in 1952, and Dr. Howery in 1954. Further investigation and advancement of breast ultrasound was carried out by Dr. Jellins, Dr. Reeves, and Dr. Kossoff in Australia; Dr. Kelly-Fry, Dr. Goldberg, and Dr. Cole-Beuglet in the United States; Dr. Wells in England; and Dr. Kobayashi in Japan. Manufacturers, in cooperation with these investigators, contributed new machines for breast ultrasound. These included prone water bath and supine water bag units.

Attempts to screen with breast ultrasound met with failure, which decreased interest in the method. Ultrasound was then limited to differentiating cystic from solid lesions.

Recently, markedly improved hand-held, electronically focused, linear array transducers have been introduced. Pioneered by Acoustic Imaging, these transducers significantly improve the quality of near-field images, which is essential in small parts imaging. Although there has been a resurgence in interest in breast ultrasound, this development has been overlooked by many who would benefit most from it. These transducers have the ability to reveal the nonmalignant patterns of breast tissue in palpable lumps. Characterizing benign lesions is invaluable to the clinician, for whom palpable lumps are a common finding.

Resistance to using ultrasound for more than cyst vs. solid differentiation continues in spite of these improvements in ultrasound's clinical usefulness. This resistance is at least partly due to the fact that, although mammographers have demanded the best and most up-to-date dedicated mammography equipment, they usually settle for the least up-to-date ultrasound equipment. Requirements similar to those for state-of-the-art mammography equipment should also be applied to ultrasound equipment, ensuring the highest quality in both areas.

Diagnostic breast ultrasound and ultrasound-guided breast biopsy are discussed in detail in Chapter 13.

PERCUTANEOUS AUTOMATED CORE BIOPSY

In 1987, after completing a fellowship in ultrasound under Dr. Michael Manco-Johnson and Dr. Delores Pretorius at the University of Colorado Health Sciences Center, a young interventional radiologist at Fitzsimons Army Medical Center, Dr. Steve Parker, began investigating the ultrasound diagnosis of prostate disease. When an automated biopsy device was introduced for prostate core biopsy, Dr. Parker began to use it in other anatomic sites, including the abdomen, thorax, and even brain (18). It was felt that this device might also be used in the breast with either stereotactic mammographic or ultrasound guidance.

Two studies of 102 patients each, carried out with the surgical group at Fitzsimons, refined the automated core-biopsy technique in the breast (19,20). In these studies all nonpalpable lesions were first stereotactically core biopsied at Radiology Imaging Associates' Breast Diagnostic and Counseling Centre in Englewood, Colorado. They were then stereotactically localized with a guide wire and excised by the Fitzsimons surgeons in the usual fashion. The results of both biopsies (core and surgical) were compared for agreement by Fitzsimons pathologists.

The automated gun technique allowed a relatively pain-free biopsy compared to previous manual techniques. The studies were begun using 18 gauge needles, but these produced fragmented cores. Dr. Parker then tried 16 gauge needles and finally 14 gauge needles specially constructed for use in the breast. These 14 gauge needles obtained excellent cores that permitted the surgical pathologists to make confident histologic diagnoses. Dr. Parker's background in ultrasound and interventional techniques allowed him to progress to an

ultrasound-guided biopsy similar to the stereotactic biopsy (21). Now the availability of stereotactic mammographic and/or ultrasound guidance permits percutaneous access to virtually any visualized breast lesion.

THE FUTURE

Where might radiology go from here? As a true screening method, mammography has serious limitations, not the least of which are radiation exposure, cost, and time expenditure. A self-directed method that patients perform on a regular basis in their own homes could be less expensive and more fruitful than mammography and could demand less time of highly qualified professionals. Research into such self-directed health care is long overdue.

New imaging methods have been tried over the years. Most investigators have focused on thermography and microwave thermography, diaphanography (light scan), computed tomography (CT) with and without contrast, ultrasound, and most recently magnetic resonance imaging (MRI). Today, ultrasound shows the greatest usefulness, but MRI, especially with gadolinium enhancement, also has promise.

New methods of staging with imaging and/or monoclonal antibodies, especially applied to lymph nodes, should be emphasized. Perhaps MRI or ultrasound will offer this opportunity. Magnetic resonance imaging with spectroscopy may prove useful in assessing lymph node status (see Chapter 14). Both stereotactic mammography and ultrasound are already being used to guide presurgical lymph node biopsy (see Chapters 8 and 12).

It has always seemed a bit incongruous for radiologists to localize and now percutaneously biopsy small, nonpalpable lesions under direct visualization and then ask surgeons to excise blindly those positive for cancer. Perhaps radiologists, in conjunction with their surgical and oncologic colleagues, will find new ways to treat these small, early cancers under direct visualization. Potential image-guided treatment modalities include laser, thermal treatment (either freezing or heating), chemoablation with agents such as absolute alcohol, directed isotope treatment using monoclonal antibodies, or percutaneous excision.

CONCLUSION

The field of breast imaging and diagnosis has a long, significant history. The research in this field has convincingly demonstrated that breast cancer mortality can be reduced through early detection and treatment. This fact makes breast imaging and breast cancer diagnosis an extremely exciting and fulfilling pursuit. This pursuit is enhanced and streamlined with the techniques described in this book. Doubtless, there are many more exciting developments to come.

REFERENCES

1. Hoeffken W, Lanyi M. *Mammography*. Philadelphia: WB Saunders; 1977.
2. Halstead WS. The results of operation for cure of cancer of the breast performed at John's Hopkins Hospital June 1889–January 1894. *Johns Hopkins Med J* 1894–5;4:297.
3. Haagensen CW. *Diseases of the breast*. 2nd ed. Philadelphia: WB Saunders; 1971.
4. Salomon A. Bertrage zur pathologie und klinic der mammakarzinome. *Arch Klin Chir* 1913;101:573–668.
5. Kleinschmidt, O. In: Zweifel-Payr: *Klinik der bosartigen Geschwulste*. Bd. IV. Leipzig: Hirzel; 1927.
6. Leborgne R. *The breast in roentgen diagnosis*. Montevideo, Uruguay: Impresora; 1953.
7. Egan RL. *Breast imaging: diagnosis and morphology of breast diseases*. Philadelphia: WB Saunders; 1988.
8. Wolfe JN. *Xeroradiography of the breast*. Springfield, IL: Charles C Thomas; 1972.
9. Gallagher HS, Martin JE. The study of mammary cancer by mammography and whole organ sectioning. *Cancer* 1969;24:1170–1178.
10. Gallagher HS, Martin JE. An orientation to the concept of minimal breast cancer. *Cancer* 1971;28:1505–1507.
11. Gershon-Cohen J, Berger SM. Mastography. *Radiol Clin North Am* 1963;1(1):115–143.
12. Ingleby H, Gershon-Cohen J. *Comparative anatomy, pathology, and roentgenology of the breast*. Philadelphia: University of Pennsylvania Press; 1960.
13. Bailer JC. Mammography: contrary view. *Ann Intern Med* 1976; 84:77–84.
14. Strax P, Venet L, Shapiro S. Value of mammography in reduction of mortality from breast cancer in mass screening. *AJR Am J Roentgenol* 1973;117:685–689.
15. Tabar L, et al. The Swedish two county trial of mammographic screening for breast cancer—recent results and calculation of benefit. *J Epidemiol Community Health* 1989;43:107–114.
16. Dodd GD, Fry K, Delany W. Pre-op localization of occult carcinoma of the breast. In: Nealon TF, ed. *Management of the patient with breast cancer*. Philadelphia: WB Saunders; 1965: 88–113.
17. Bulmgren J, Jacobson B, Nordenstrom B. Stereotaxis instrument for needle biopsy of the mamma. *AJR Am J Roentgenol* 1977;129:121–125.
18. Parker SH, Hopper KD, Yakes WF, Gibson MD, Ownbey JL, Carter TE. Image-directed percutaneous biopsies with a biopsy gun. *Radiology* 1989;171:663–669.
19. Parker SH, Lovin JD, Jobe WE, et al. Stereotactic breast biopsy with a biopsy gun. *Radiology* 1990;176:741–747.
20. Parker SH, Lovin JD, Jobe WE, Burke BJ, Hopper KD, Yakes WF. Nonpalpable breast lesions: stereotactic automated large-core biopsies. *Radiology* 1991;180:403–407.
21. Parker SH, Jobe WE, Dennis MA, et al. Ultrasound-guided automated large core breast biopsy. *Radiology* [*in press*].

Percutaneous Breast Biopsy, edited by
Steve H. Parker and William E. Jobe.
Raven Press, Ltd., New York © 1993.

CHAPTER 2

Needle Selection

Steve H. Parker

Many needles are available for use in percutaneous breast biopsy. Although none are dedicated breast biopsy needles, these generic needles are used for diagnosing breast disease. Two categories exist: small-gauge (20 to 23 gauge), or *fine-needles*, and large-gauge (14 to 18 gauge) or *core needles*. Both fine-needles and core needles can be used either manually or in automated biopsy guns.

FINE-NEEDLES

Small-gauge needles are classified by the needle-tip configuration. The conventional spinal needle was the original "skinny" needle and is still sometimes used for breast biopsy. The Chiba needle, a slightly modified spinal needle with a beveled tip, is one of the more widely used fine-needles. Other commonly used fine-needles include the Franzeen, which has a serrated tip, and the Turner, which has a cutting surface about the circumference of its tip.

With most fine-needles, aspiration is applied during the procedure; thus, the name *fine-needle aspiration biopsy* (FNAB). A FNAB is usually performed manually, using a 21 to 23 gauge needle with a syringe attached. After the needle is placed in the desired location, vacuum is created and the operator moves the needle up and down to collect cellular material. Three or more passes are usually made. Smears are fixed and stained on glass slides. If a cytopathologist attends the biopsy, a preliminary cytologic diagnosis can be made from microscopic evaluation of the smears.

Fine-needle aspiration biopsy is discussed in detail in Chapter 9.

CORE NEEDLES

Most large-gauge, core needles are of the Tru-cut design, which consists of an inner trocar with a sample notch at its distal end and an outer cutting cannula. During operation, the trocar portion is pushed forward first and tissue is collected within the sample notch. Then the outer cutting cannula is pushed forward, shearing off the sample from the surrounding tissue and enclosing it within the walls of the cannula.

Since most radiologists have focused on FNAB, they have largely ignored large-gauge needles for percutaneous breast biopsy. Surgeons, however, often manually biopsy palpable breast lesions with large (usually 14 gauge Tru-cut) needles. Surgeons are generally more confident of these diagnoses than of those from FNAB because the large needles provide tissue that can be analyzed histologically in the same way as surgical specimens.

Manual biopsy with 14 gauge Tru-cut needles has disadvantages, however. The procedure requires two hands and some level of experience. Manual insertion makes it possible for the needle to slide off of or away from very firm or fibrotic lesions. Lesions, such as fibroadenomas, that move rather freely in the loose fatty/connective tissue of the breast can also be pushed out of the path of a manually advanced needle.

The introduction of the Bard Biopty gun in the mid 1980s (Fig. 1) dramatically changed needle biopsy, especially in the breast. The rapid action of automated devices overcame the drawbacks of manually operated Tru-cut needles. Biopsy guns obtain tissue with split-second sampling when the operator merely pushes a button. Tissue acquisition is automatic and consistent so the operator can concentrate his or her full attention on accurate targeting. Rapidly fired needles can penetrate very firm and/or fibrotic lesions, as well as mobile lesions before they slip out of the way. Automated biopsy devices also decrease patient discomfort because

S.H. Parker: Radiology Imaging Associates, Breast Diagnostic and Counseling Centre, Englewood, Colorado 80111.

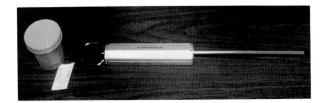

FIG. 1. Bard Biopty gun with case closed. A sterile specimen cup with a small amount of physiologic saline is adjacent to the gun.

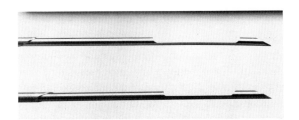

FIG. 2. Comparison of the sample notches of two 14 gauge needles. The sample notch of the top 14 gauge needle is slightly deeper and longer than the notch of the bottom needle. (Courtesy of Geoffrey Wheeler.)

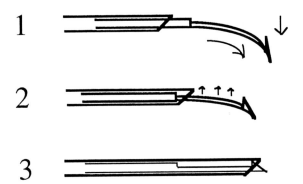

FIG. 3. Schematic representation of the desired diving action of the trocar portion of the needle actively trapping tissue within the notch, rather than relying on passive prolapse of tissue into the notch. **1:** As the trocar is projected forward, it dives somewhat. **2:** The cannula then projects forward, and, because it is stiffer than the flexible sample notch, it pulls the sample notch back up. **3:** This shears off a full core.

the biopsy is faster than manual biopsy. The cores obtained with automated biopsy guns have better quality and integrity than have manually obtained specimens (1,2).

The first attempts to combine core needles and biopsy guns for use in the breast were made with 18 gauge or 20 gauge needles and short-throw (1.15-cm excursion) biopsy guns (3,4). Specimens obtained with 18 gauge and 20 gauge needles were not entirely satisfactory, however, and short-excursion automated biopsy devices were inferior to the long-excursion variety. The eventual combination of 14 gauge needles and long-throw (2.3-cm excursion) biopsy guns produced a percutaneous biopsy as accurate as surgical biopsy (5,6).

Several different manufacturers now make 14 gauge, Tru-cut needles that can fit into the Bard Biopty gun and its imitators. Since all biopsy guns operate very similarly, using spring-loaded sleds onto which the trocar and cannula hubs of the biopsy needle are placed, there is not much difference among them. Again, the long-throw versions are superior to the short-throw guns. Unlike the guns, however, core needles designed for biopsy guns can differ markedly in their performance, despite the fact that they may superficially look the same.

Several characteristics must be carefully evaluated when selecting a core needle. The length and depth of the sample notch are of primary importance. A longer and deeper sample notch naturally will acquire more tissue than a shorter more shallow sample notch, even in the same gauge needle (Fig. 2). The flexibility of the distal aspect of the trocar portion of the needle where the sample notch resides is also important. The more flexible the steel is here, the better. A flexible trocar dives slightly more than a stiffer one. This diving action is necessary to obtain a high-quality core (Fig. 3). Manually bending the trocar portion slightly in the same direction as the bevel can enhance this diving motion if adequate tissue is not obtained on the initial passes (Fig. 4). Finally, the sharpness of the needle should be considered. The point of the trocar tip and the cutting portion of the cannula should be exquisitely sharp. The trocar-point sharpness determines how easily the biopsy needle glides through firm, fibrous septae and areas of fibrocystic change. If the trocar point is not sharp, the needle may merely push firm tissue, along with the lesion behind it, ahead of the needle. Sharper cannulas deliver cleaner, more consistent cores, without crush artifact.

If the core needle is selected carefully with attention to the above-mentioned details, then the quality, quantity, and consistency of the biopsy specimens should be excellent. Even if the localization is performed perfectly, core biopsy will not be successful if a substand-

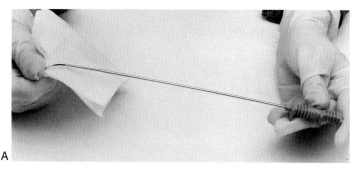
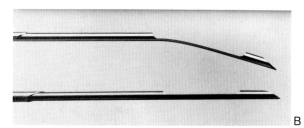

A   B

FIG. 4. A: Manual bending of the sample notch portion of the trocar to enhance the quantity of tissue acquisition. **B:** View of needle after bending. (Courtesy of Geoffrey Wheeler.)

ard needle fails to acquire adequate tissue for a firm diagnosis.

Automated large-core biopsy is discussed in detail in Chapters 7 (using stereotactic guidance) and 13 (using ultrasound guidance).

FINE-NEEDLE ASPIRATION BIOPSY VS. CORE BIOPSY

There has been considerable debate over the relative merits of FNAB and core biopsy in the breast, as well as elsewhere in the body. This debate has largely been resolved in favor of automated core biopsy in virtually all anatomic sites except the breast. Most likely, breast biopsy will eventually follow the lead of biopsy in other anatomic sites, and automated core biopsy will become the method of choice.

Breast FNAB is likely to be unsuccessful at many institutions because cytopathology, a difficult art and science, often is not available in its highest form (7–9) (see Chapter 3). Fine-needle aspiration biopsy requires a cytopathologist or cytotechnologist attending the biopsy to ensure proper handling of the specimen. Ideally, the cytopathologist confirms adequate tissue sampling at the time of the biopsy and can conceivably make the diagnosis immediately with preliminary microscopic evaluation. However, this increases the cost of the procedure, and preliminary diagnoses are occa-

sionally changed after further evaluation of all of the permanently fixed specimens is completed.

In addition, FNAB has insufficient tissue rates as high as 37% (8), false-negative rates as high as 31% (8), occasional false-positive results, and inconclusive diagnoses of both malignant and benign lesions. Many breast surgeons will not rely on the results of FNAB because of these drawbacks, and patients frequently are subjected to surgical biopsy anyway. Thus, FNAB is often an unnecessary layer of testing and additional cost.

Automated large-core biopsy overcomes many of the drawbacks of FNAB. First, insufficient tissue is rarely, if ever, a problem because the core tissue is easily visible to the naked eye (Fig. 5). The radiologist does not need a pathologist to verify the specimens' adequacy. If visibly adequate tissue is not obtained, another pass can always be made. Second, large-core gun biopsies theoretically decrease false-negative results because they obtain larger quantities of tissue per pass. Third, no cases of false-positive diagnoses on permanent section have been reported with core biopsy.

Most importantly, the histologic analysis of core tissue renders definitive benign and malignant diagnoses (unlike the inconclusive diagnoses, such as "no malignancy present," made with cytologic aspirate). Complete benign diagnoses like "fibrocystic mastopathy" (Fig. 6), "pericanalicular fibroadenoma" (Fig. 7), or "sclerosing adenosis" (Fig. 8) can be obtained from core samples. Fine-needle aspiration biopsy frequently cannot distinguish between false negatives due to sampling error and true negatives such as fibroadenomas. Thus, with the definitive benign diagnoses made with core biopsy, surgical biopsy can be confidently avoided.

Histologic evaluation of core tissue can also definitively differentiate between *in situ* and invasive carcinoma, which cytology cannot. Not knowing whether a cancer is invasive complicates and potentially length-

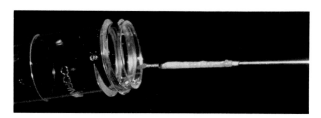

FIG. 5. Sample notch of a 14 gauge needle filled almost entirely with breast tissue.

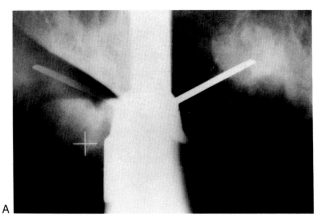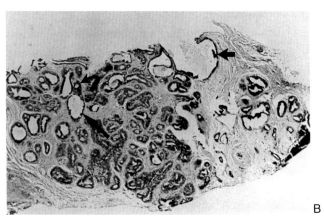

A

B

FIG. 6. Fibrocystic change. **A:** Stereotactic views of asymmetric density with the needle in the prefire position. **B:** Photomicrograph of the gun core demonstrating elements of fibrocystic change: ductal ectasia (*long arrow*), ductal hyperplasia (*curved arrow*), and papillomatosis (*short arrow*). (From Parker et al., Ref. *3*, with permission.)

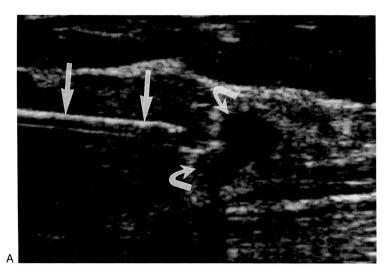

A

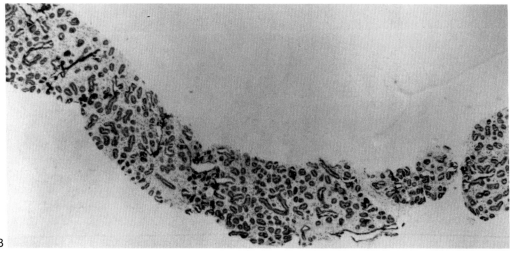

B

FIG. 7. Pericanalicular fibroadenoma. **A:** Ultrasound image showing a biopsy needle (*long arrows*) at the periphery of a hypoechoic lesion (*curved arrows*) in the prefire position. **B:** Low-power photomicrograph of a gun core diagnostic of pericanalicular fibroadenoma.

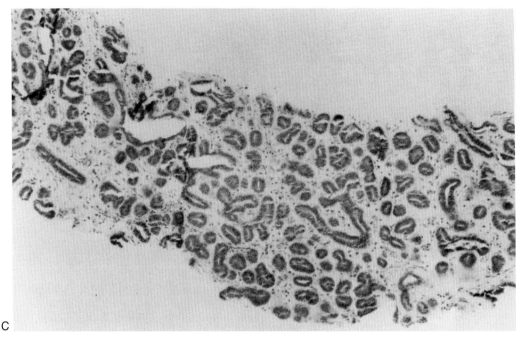

FIG. 7. (*Continued*) **C:** High-power photomicrograph of the same lesion. (From Parker and Jobe, Ref. 9a, with permission.)

ens the definitive surgical procedure (10) (Fig. 9). Classifying malignant neoplasms with core biopsy facilitates appropriate treatment planning in one stage (Fig. 10).

Theoretically, large-gauge needles might increase morbidity (11,12). Perhaps this explains why radiologists have avoided using them in the breast. The techniques of FNAB were applied to the breast before more widespread acceptance of core biopsy elsewhere in the body. Naturally, investigators used needles and tech-

niques honed during their experience in other areas of the body. Radiologists apparently failed to consider that the breast is virtually devoid of vital structures. The loose connective tissue of the breast is not susceptible to significant injury even with large-gauge needles. In over 1,000 core biopsies performed with 14 gauge needles at the Breast Diagnostic and Counseling Centre, Englewood, Colorado, no significant hematoma or infection has occurred. A similar lack of significant complications has been reported elsewhere (6)

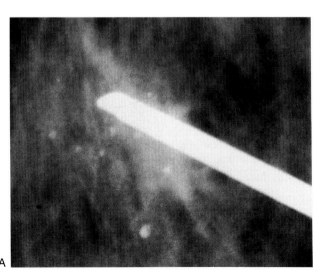

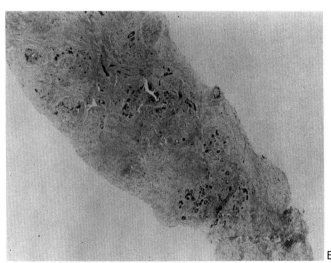

FIG. 8. Sclerosing adenosis. **A:** Postfire view from one stereotactic image after the needle has traversed the calcifications. **B:** Photomicrograph of gun core definitively diagnosing sclerosing adenosis.

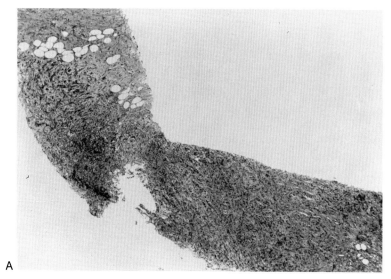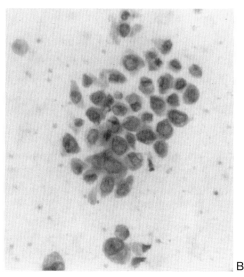

A B

FIG. 9. Comparison of 14 gauge core and FNAB. **A:** Photomicrograph of 14 gauge core diagnostic of infiltrating ductal carcinoma. **B** Cytologic specimen showing malignant cells without the ability to determine invasiveness. (From Parker and Jobe, Ref. 9a, with permission.)

(personal communications: Fred Burbank, M.D.; Peter Dempsey, M.D.; Phil Evans, M.D.; William Hutchins, M.D.; Mary Lechner, M.D.).

Although some physicians use small-gauge needles with automated biopsy guns in the breast (4), these procedures cannot be considered true core biopsies because small needles usually harvest only scanty specimens that are not significantly different from those gathered by FNAB. At best they obtain tissue fragments, but their quality virtually never matches that gathered by large-gauge, core-biopsy needles.

Older reports comparing aspiration needles with core-biopsy needles in the breast gave conflicting results (13–16). Although some investigators found FNAB to be superior to core biopsy, their studies are subject to skepticism because they compared multiple skinny-needle passes to only one manual core-needle pass. In addition, they performed manual freehand, "blind" biopsy [i.e., *without* automated biopsy instruments or image guidance (stereotactic or ultrasound)]. They also failed to address the inability of FNAB to render definitive benign diagnoses, an important consideration in breast biopsy, as the vast majority of lesions sampled are benign.

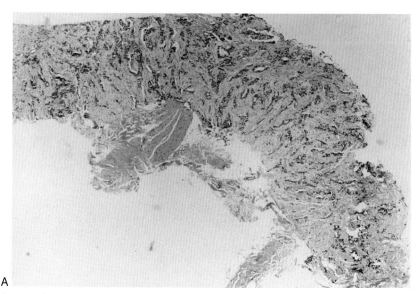

A

FIG. 10. Comparison of 14 gauge core and surgical specimens. **A:** Photomicrograph of core demonstrating infiltrating ductal carcinoma.

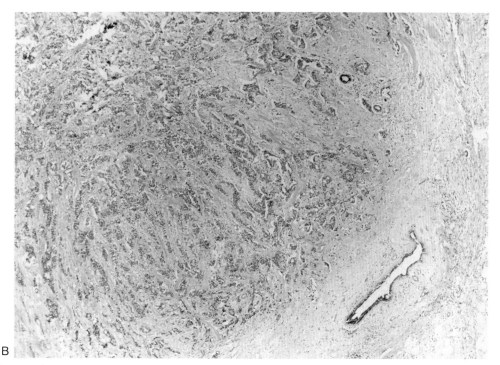

FIG. 10. (*Continued*) **B:** Surgical excisional specimen showing the exact same architecture. Thus, core diagnosis can be acted upon with the same degree of certainty as with surgical excisional diagnosis. (From Parker et al., Ref. 10a, with permission.)

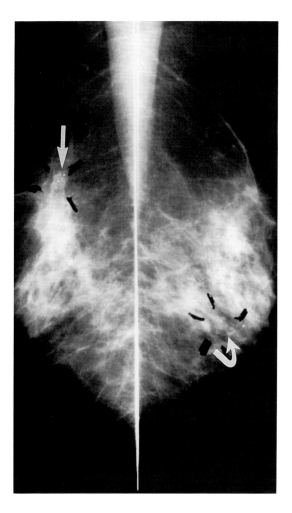

FIG. 11. Patient with a cluster of microcalcifications in each breast. Both clusters were stereotactically biopsied. One cluster (*straight arrow*) was diagnosed as a degenerated fibroadenoma, and the other (*curved arrow*) as infiltrating ductal carcinoma. Therapeutic attention could then be directed to the cluster representing malignancy, and the other cluster was left alone. If these had been biopsied with the FNAB technique, however, with one answer "malignancy" and the other "no evidence of malignancy," most surgeons would excise the benign cluster as well as the malignant neoplasm because of the uncertainty surrounding the nebulous FNAB diagnosis.

FUTURE DEVELOPMENTS

Other large-core needles besides the Tru-cut will probably be forthcoming. Work is in progress to develop a new full-core cannula needle that will acquire more tissue for a given needle diameter than does the Tru-cut variety. Existing full-core cannula needles that rely on vacuum to obtain their core do not seem to work reliably. New designs will focus on assuring reliable tissue acquisition.

Other devices being developed will acquire even larger specimens percutaneously. These devices, classified as minimal excisional biopsy devices rather than as incisional core-biopsy needles, would theoretically be more likely to produce mammographic pseudolesions and poor cosmesis.

CONCLUSION

Fourteen gauge needles most consistently provide the highest quality, intact cores in breast tissue (5). Automated guns are preferred because they are easy to use, decrease patient discomfort, and improve specimen quality compared to manually operated 14 gauge needles (1). The long-throw guns are superior to the short-throw variety (1,3,4).

Perceptions are changing across the United States regarding the best needle selection for breast biopsy (and biopsy of other anatomic sites, as well). More physicians are recognizing the drawbacks of FNAB and the advantages of histologic core biopsy (Fig. 11). As a result, radiologists stand on the edge of a global change in how breast biopsy is performed.

REFERENCES

1. Hopper KD, Baird DE, Reddy VV, et al. Efficacy of automated biopsy guns versus conventional biopsy needles in the pygmy pig. *Radiology* 1990;176:671–676.
2. Parker SH, Hopper KD, Yakes WF, Gibson MD, Ownbey JL, Carter TE. Image-directed percutaneous biopsies with a biopsy gun. *Radiology* 1989;171:663–669.
3. Parker SH, Lovin JD, Jobe WE, et al. Stereotactic breast biopsy with a biopsy gun. *Radiology* 1990;176:741–747.
4. Dowlatshahi K, Yaremko ML, Kluskens LF, Jokich PM. Nonpalpable breast lesions: findings of stereotaxic needle-core biopsy and fine-needle aspiration cytology. *Radiology* 1991;181:745–750.
5. Parker SH, Lovin JD, Jobe WE, Burke BJ, Hopper KD, Yakes WF. Nonpalpable breast lesions: stereotactic automated large-core biopsies. *Radiology* 1991;180:403–407.
6. Myer JE. Value of large-core biopsy of occult breast lesions. *AJR Am J Roentgenol* 1992;158:991–992.
7. Dowlatshahi K, Gent HJ, Schmidt R, Jokich PM, Bibbo M, Sprenger E. Nonpalpable breast tumors: diagnosis with stereotaxic localization and fine-needle aspiration. *Radiology* 1989;170:427–433.
8. Grant GS, Goellner JR, Welch JS, Martin JK. Fine-needle aspiration of the breast. *Mayo Clin Proc* 1986;61:377–381.
9. Sundaram M, Wolverson MK, Heiberg E, Pilla T, Vas WG, Shields JB. Utility of CT-guided abdominal aspiration procedures. *AJR Am J Roentgenol* 1982;139:1111–1115.
9a. Parker SH, Jobe WE. Large-core biopsy offers reliable diagnosis. *Diagn Imaging* 1990;12(10):93.
10. Lofgren M, Andersson I, Lindholm K. Stereotactic fine-needle aspiration for cytologic diagnosis of nonpalpable breast lesions. *AJR Am J Roentgenol* 1990;154:1191–1195.
10a. Parker SH, Jobe WE, Dennis MA, et al. Ultrasound-guided automated large core breast biopsy. *Radiology* 1993;187:507–511.
11. Charboneau JW, Reading CC, Welch TJ. CT and sonographically guided needle biopsy: current techniques and new innovations. *AJR Am J Roentgenol* 1990;154:1–10.
12. Gazelle GS, Haaga JR. Guided percutaneous biopsy of intraabdominal lesions. *AJR Am J Roentgenol* 1989;153:929–935.
13. Elston CW, Cotton RE, Davies DJ, Blamey RW. A comparison of the use of the "Tru-Cut" needle and fine needle aspiration cytology in the preoperative diagnosis of carcinoma of the breast. *Histopathology* 1978;2:239–254.
14. Vorherr H. Breast aspiration biopsy with multihole needles for histologic and cytologic examination. *Am J Obstet Gynecol* 1985;151:70–76.
15. Pederson L, Guldhammer B, Kamby C, Aasted M, Rose C. Fine needle aspiration and Tru-Cut biopsy in the diagnosis of soft tissue metastases in breast cancer. *Eur J Cancer Clin Oncol* 1986;22:1045–1052.
16. Shabot MM, Goldberg IM, Schick P, Nieberg R, Pilch YH. Aspiration cytology is superior to Tru-Cut needle biopsy in establishing the diagnosis of clinically suspicious breast masses. *Ann Surg* 1982;196:122–126.

Percutaneous Breast Biopsy, edited by
Steve H. Parker and William E. Jobe.
Raven Press, Ltd., New York © 1993.

CHAPTER 3

The Pathologist's Perspective

John E. Truell and Peter J. Philpott

The pathologic evaluation of mammographic and ultra-sonographic abnormalities of the breast sampled by a large-core automated biopsy has several goals. These goals are to provide definitive diagnoses of both benign and malignant processes with a greater degree of sensitivity and specificity than is available with currently used procedures such as FNAB and to permit modifications of clinical management based on these diagnoses. Comparing FNAB and large-core automated biopsy from a pathologist's perspective can help assess whether or not these goals are realized.

FINE-NEEDLE ASPIRATION BIOPSY WITH CYTOLOGIC INTERPRETATION

The preoperative evaluation of breast abnormalities has been the subject of much interest and numerous articles. Many articles published during the past decade attempting to define the utility of fine-needle aspiration biopsy with cytologic interpretation of nonpalpable breast masses described several of the problems commonly encountered with this procedure. In all of these series, fine-needle aspiration of breast masses showed a significant lack of sensitivity (i.e., a negative cytologic result in a subsequently proven cancer) (1–6). A number of series reported a small but significant lack of specificity (i.e., a positive cytologic result with a subsequent benign biopsy) (1–3). The reasons that FNAB failed to produce a definitive diagnosis include the following:

1. Most pathologists, primarily trained in surgical pathology with limited training in cytology, are more comfortable with histologic preparations (1).
2. In centers where radical surgery may follow a cytologic diagnosis of malignancy, pathologists are jus-

tifiably very conservative and cautious, thereby potentially underdiagnosing malignancy.
3. Sampling errors are relatively common with some breast lesions (2). Densely fibrotic masses, small tumors, and the experience of the operator are all variables contributing to inadequate samples.
4. A number of benign processes may demonstrate cellular changes in a cytologic preparation, leading to equivocal interpretations. These processes include but are not limited to fibroadenomas, sclerosing adenosis, and variations of ductal hyperplasia.
5. A number of malignant tumors do not lend themselves to diagnosis by cytologic means (2,7). These include tubular carcinoma, infiltrating and *in situ* lobular carcinomas, and ductal carcinomas made up of small cells.
6. Distinguishing *in situ* from invasive malignancy is not possible with cytology.

Many pathologists remain skeptical of the utility of FNAB because of its understandable but inherent lack of sensitivity and because of inadequate samples. Many pathologists require frozen section confirmation of any positive cytologic diagnosis, and most negative cytologic diagnoses are soon followed by open biopsy. Whether this is an effective use of time and money is open to debate.

AUTOMATED LARGE-CORE BIOPSY

Stereotactic or ultrasound-guided large-core biopsy permits the assessment of histologic as well as cytologic findings. Therefore, this procedure solves many of the problems encountered with fine-needle aspiration biopsy.

Depending on the nature of the breast tissue sampled, the characteristics of large-core biopsy specimens may vary from quite friable and fragmented to

J.E. Truell and P.J. Philpott: Department of Pathology, Swedish Medical Center, Englewood, Colorado 80110.

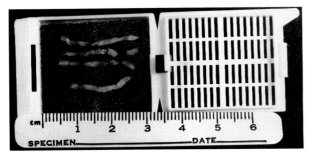

FIG. 1. Close-up photograph of a plastic tissue cassette with a sponge in the bottom and breast needle biopsy material placed on the sponge.

single, very firm, and cohesive pieces up to 20 to 30 mm long. Because unfixed tissue is susceptible to crush artifact and to drying, it must be handled gently and fixed rapidly in standard 10% formalin. The formalin container with tissue may be kept at room temperature and must be protected from freezing if transported.

Specimens received through the Pathology Department of Swedish Medical Center (Englewood, Colorado) are processed with the following method. All biopsy fragments from the same anatomic site are received in one container and processed by placing the tissue pieces between sponges (S/P Brand foam biopsy pads; Baxter Scientific Products, McGaw Park, Illinois) in a single plastic cassette (Tissue-Tek Uni-Cassette; Miles Inc., Elkhart, Indiana) (Fig. 1). The tissue

is processed routinely through the standard dehydration and infiltration steps to paraffin. Each piece is embedded in a separate block, with care taken during this embedding process to lay each piece flat along its entire length to allow sectioning of the entire piece. Serial sections of each block are made sufficient to yield six or eight separate sections on each slide, depending on the size of the individual pieces (Fig. 2). The stain used is hematoxylin and eosin (H&E).

Calcification (calcium phosphate or hydroxyapatite) is usually visible in the routine slides. Thus, special stains for calcium are not performed. If the biopsy is being done for calcification and no calcium is seen, the slides are viewed by polarized illumination to search for calcium oxalate (8,9). Some calcifications seen on specimen radiography and viewed with polarized light may still not be seen on histopathology. Reasons for this include microtome loss and calcifications residing in a different section of the block.

The pathology report indicates the presence or absence of breast tissue proper and then describes and diagnoses any lesion seen. The same pathologic criteria applied to standard surgical biopsy specimens are used. In over 500 specimens resulting from this procedure examined at Swedish Medical Center, only one was unsatisfactory because of insufficient material. The remaining specimens were all sufficient for a definitive malignant or benign diagnosis. Malignant diagnoses included invasive ductal carcinoma, tubular car-

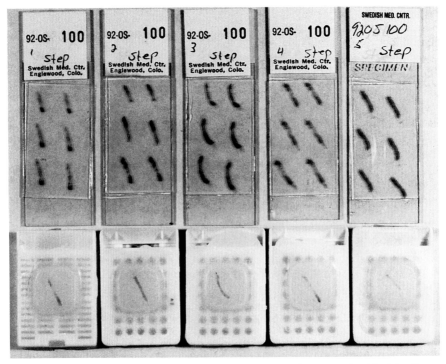

FIG. 2. Close-up photograph of a set of slides made from tissue embedded in the respective paraffin blocks. (H&E)

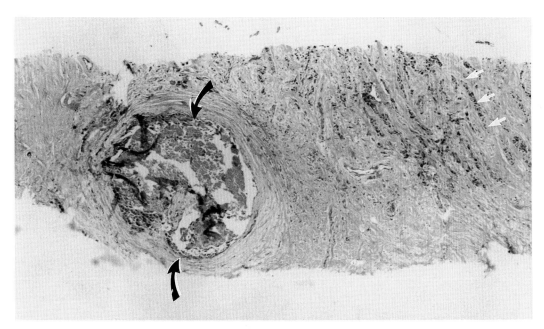

FIG. 3. Photomicrograph of comedo carcinoma. Note the intraductal component (*curved arrows*) and the adjacent infiltrating cords of cells (*small arrows*). (Original magnification ×100)

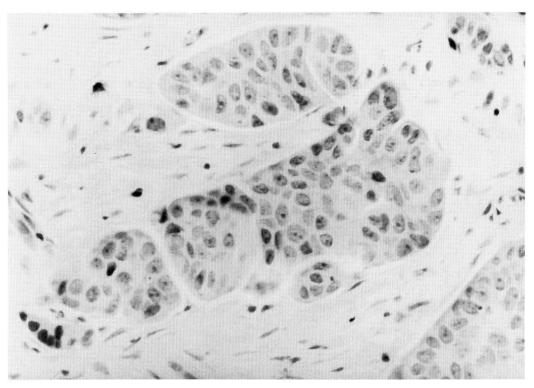

FIG. 4. Photomicrograph of nests of infiltrating ductal carcinoma cells. Note the well-preserved histologic and cytologic detail, including variable numbers of nucleoli in tumor-cell nuclei best seen centrally. (Original magnification, ×400)

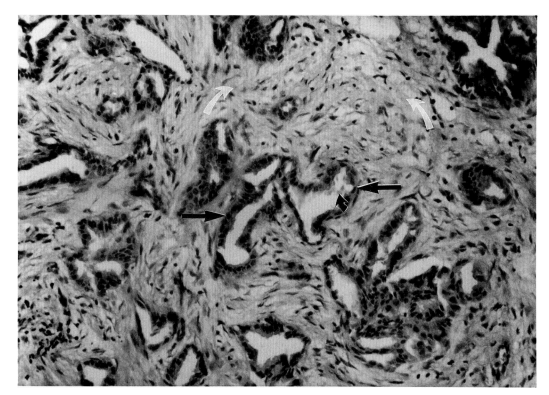

FIG. 5. Photomicrograph of tubular carcinoma. Note the desmoplastic stroma (*curved arrows*) surrounding irregularly shaped tubular structures (*straight arrows*). The tubules are lined by a single layer of well-differentiated cells with prominent "apocrine snouts" on the luminal surfaces of the cells (*small curved arrow*). (Original magnification ×400)

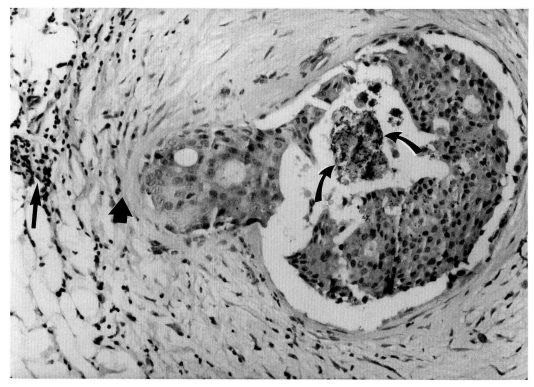

FIG. 6. Photomicrograph of a duct involved by comedo carcinoma (*in situ*). There is necrotic detritus in the duct (*curved arrows*), prominent periductal fibrosis (*arrowhead*), and chronic inflammation (*straight arrow*). (Original magnification ×400)

cinoma, invasive lobular carcinoma, and mucinous (colloid) carcinoma (Figs. 3 to 5). Intraductal (*in situ*) carcinomas included comedo (Fig. 6), cribriform (Fig. 7), and papillary carcinomas. Necrosis, nuclear grade, and type of calcifications could be determined in these cases. Hyperplasia could be divided into atypical ductal hyperplasia (Fig. 8), hyperplasia of the usual (typical) type, and lobular hyperplasia. No case diagnosed as a malignant neoplasm was later found not to be malignant. (There were no false positives).

The largest single category of a benign process was fibrocystic mastopathy or the fibrosclerosis variant of fibrocystic mastopathy. These biopsies demonstrated a wide spectrum of histologic features of fibrocystic mastopathy but did not demonstrate significant epithelial hyperplasia. Adenosis (sclerosing and microglandular forms) were generally included with the fibrocystic mastopathy category (Figs. 9 and 10). The second most common benign diagnosis was fibroadenoma (Fig. 11), with one case diagnosed as a phyllodes tumor (Fig. 12). Other benign processes included chronic mastitis, nonspecific calcification, lactational change, an intramammary lymph node (Fig. 13), fat necrosis, and lipoma.

If automated large-core biopsy is to be more clinically useful than fine-needle aspiration, two goals should be achieved. The first is to provide definitive diagnoses of infiltrating carcinoma and carcinoma *in situ*. The second is to provide a definitive diagnosis of benign processes, which in most instances would preclude an open biopsy. Additional information such as estrogen and progesterone receptor status, DNA ploidy, and S-phase percentage may be obtained from the paraffin-embedded tissue. (DNA ploidy and S-phase percentage are determined by cytometric analysis.) Other prognostic markers may also be evaluated. All of this information may be useful in planning definitive therapy.

All of the automated core-biopsy specimens diagnosed at Swedish Medical Center as infiltrating ductal carcinoma or ductal carcinoma *in situ* have been proven at the definitive surgical procedure. With the large artifact-free biopsies obtained by this procedure, one can expect 100% specificity of a positive diagnosis (or at least as close to 100% specificity as one can expect from histopathology). Three cases diagnosed on the core biopsy as atypical ductal hyperplasia were subsequently upgraded to ductal carcinoma *in situ* at the time of follow-up surgery. This would not be unexpected given the continuum of atypical hyperplasia and low-nuclear-grade ductal carcinoma *in situ* and the fact that any distinction between these two entities is as semantic as it is histologic (10). Finally, unusual carcinomas such as tubular carcinoma can be diagnosed with this procedure. Two tubular carcinomas diagnosed on core biopsy were both later proven at definitive surgery.

The major benefit of this procedure may not be in

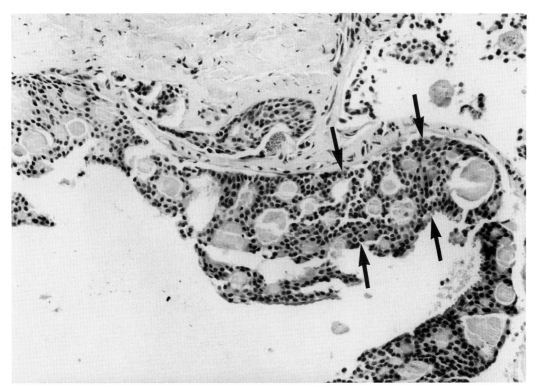

FIG. 7. Photomicrograph of a duct lined by intraductal carcinoma cells with a cribriform pattern (*straight arrows*). (Original magnification ×400)

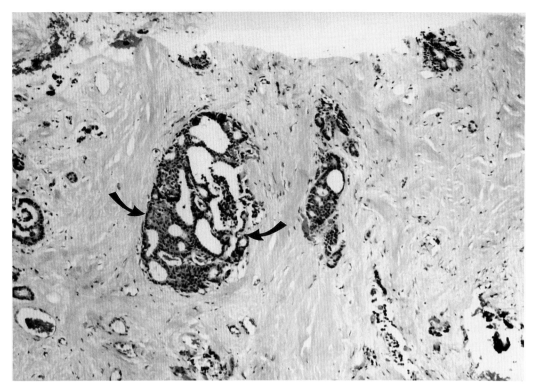

FIG. 8. Photomicrograph of a duct showing atypical intraductal hyperplasia (*curved arrows*). (Original magnification ×200)

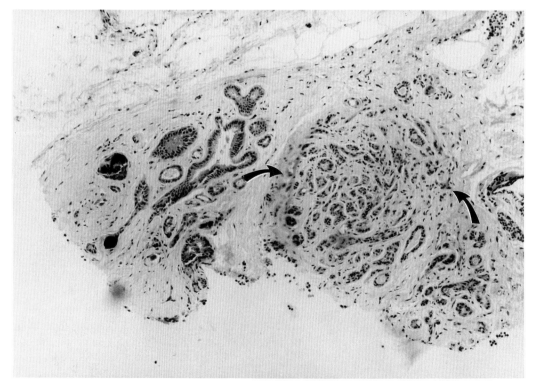

FIG. 9. Photomicrograph of fibrocystic mastopathy and a focus of sclerosing adenosis (*curved arrows*). (Original magnification ×200)

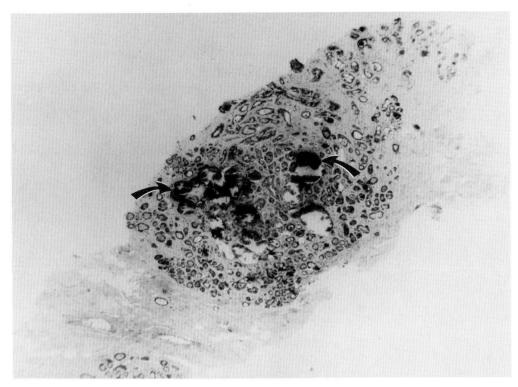

FIG. 10. Photomicrograph of an area of sclerosing adenosis with prominent dark-staining calcification (*curved arrows*). (Original magnification ×200)

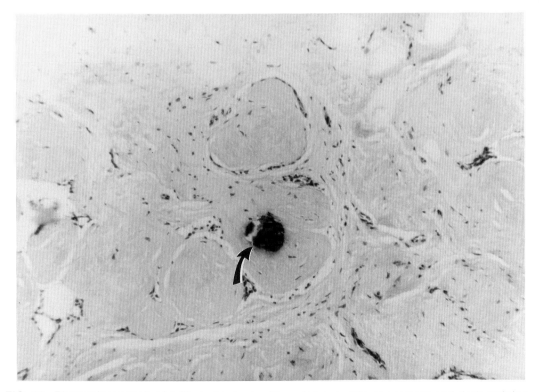

FIG. 11. Photomicrograph of a fibroadenoma with an intracanalicular pattern and dark-staining calcification (*curved arrow*). (Original magnification ×200)

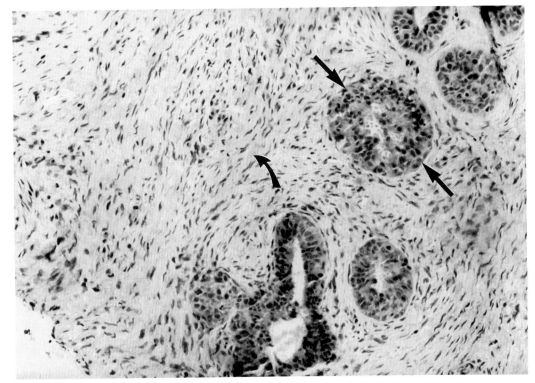

FIG. 12. Photomicrograph of benign-appearing phyllodes tumor. Note the cellular stroma (*curved arrows*) and the ductal structures lined by hyperplastic cells (*straight arrows*). (Original magnification ×400)

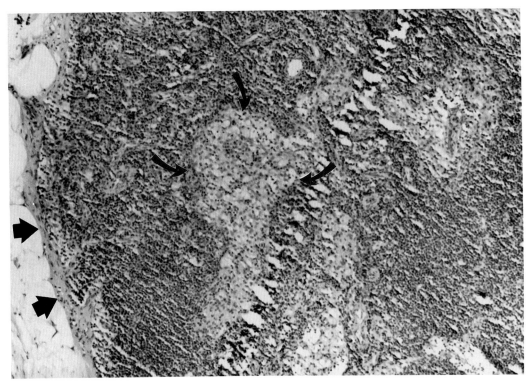

FIG. 13. Photomicrograph of a portion of an intramammary lymph node. Note the distinct capsule (*arrowheads*) and the preserved architecture with sinusoidal hyperplasia (*curved arrows*). (Original magnification ×200)

the diagnoses of malignant processes but rather in the definitive diagnoses of a variety of benign processes. Relatively common benign processes such as sclerosing adenosis, fibroadenoma, and fibrocystic mastopathy can be diagnosed with confidence. Additionally, intramammary lymph nodes, areas of fat necrosis, and previous biopsy sites can be recognized. All of these may present problems on interpretation of the cytologic features. Naturally, in the face of a highly suspicious mammogram or ultrasound image, no diagnosis should preclude open biopsy. It is therefore essential that good communication between the radiologist and the pathologist exists for adequate coordination of the biopsy findings with the mammogram or ultrasound images.

The issue of hyperplasia deserves special mention. Tissue examination permits the diagnosis of both typical and atypical ductal hyperplasia, as well as lobular hyperplasia. As mentioned above, several cases of atypical ductal hyperplasia were modified to ductal carcinoma *in situ* at subsequent surgery. It is therefore recommended that any diagnosis of atypical ductal hyperplasia be followed by open biopsy. Whether typical or mildly atypical ductal hyperplasia found in a core biopsy should be followed by open biopsy will depend on a number of factors including patient, physician, and institutional preferences. A recent article by Rosai (10) may sway more people to open biopsy after a diagnosis of hyperplasia. This article emphasized individual variation, even among recognized experts, in applying the histologic criteria of typical ductal hyperplasia, atypical ductal hyperplasia, and ductal carcinoma *in situ* (DCIS).

A final issue that must be addressed in all centers performing this procedure is the evaluation of areas of clustered calcification. Observing calcium in these specimens is not difficult. However, whether five or six core biopsies of an area of granular calcification represent an adequate sample is a legitimate question. Biopsy of dystrophic calcifications associated with higher nuclear grade DCIS should usually yield the correct diagnosis when the calcifications are included in the specimen (11). However, small areas of low-nuclear-grade ductal carcinoma *in situ* not intimately associated with the calcifications and often involving only a fraction of the biopsy specimen may be found in open surgical biopsy cases. Whether or not to perform a core biopsy on widespread calcifications that may be associated with noncomedo, low-nuclear-grade DCIS is an issue that requires future follow-up and consideration.

In summary, automated large-core breast biopsy provides a definitive diagnosis for most breast masses. The procedure can also render a histologic evaluation of such other areas of mammographic or ultrasound abnormality as areas of clustered calcification and diffuse fibrocystic change.

REFERENCES

1. Frable WJ. Needle aspiration biopsy: past, present, and future. *Hum Pathol* 1989;20:504–517.
2. Eisenberg AJ, Hajdu SI, Wilhelmus J, Melamed MR, Kinne D. Preoperative aspiration cytology of breast tumors. *Acta Cytol* 1986;30:135–146.
3. Helvie MA, Baker DE, Adler DD, Andersson I, Naylor B, Buckwalter KA. Radiographically guided fine-needle aspiration of nonpalpable breast lesions. *Radiology* 1990;174:657–661.
4. Zajicek J, Caspersson T, Jakobsson P, Kudynowski J, Linsk J, Us-Kravosek M. Cytologic diagnosis of mammary tumors from aspiration biopsy smears. *Acta Cytol* 1970;14:370–376.
5. Nicastri GR, Reed WP, Dziura BR. The accuracy of malignant diagnoses established by fine needle aspiration cytologic procedures of mammary masses. *Surg Gynecol Obstet* 1991;7:72–74.
6. Horgan PG, Waldron D, Mooney E, O'Brien D, McGuire M, Given HF. The role of aspiration cytologic examination in the diagnosis of carcinoma of the breast. *Surg Gynecol Obstet* 1991; 172:290–292.
7. Gupta RK, Dowle C. Fine-needle aspiration cytology of tubular carcinoma of the breast in a young woman. *Diagn Cytopathol* 1991;7:72–74.
8. Gonzales JEG, Caldwell RG, Vlaitis J. Calcium oxalate crystals in the breast. *Am J Surg Pathol* 1991;15:586–591.
9. Tornos C, Silva E, El-Naggar A, Pritzker KPH. Calcium oxalate crystals in breast biopsies. *Am J Surg Pathol* 1990;14:961–968.
10. Rosai J. Borderline epithelial lesions of the breast. *Am J Surg Pathol* 1991;15:209–221.
11. Holland R, Hendriks JHCL, Verbeek ALM, Mravunac M, Schuurmans Stekhoven JH. Extent, distribution, and mammographic/histological correlations of breast ductal carcinoma *in situ*. *Lancet* 1990;335:519–522.

Percutaneous Breast Biopsy, edited by
Steve H. Parker and William E. Jobe.
Raven Press, Ltd., New York © 1993.

CHAPTER 4

Nursing Considerations

Joan P. Camp

A nurse can be an important asset to a smoothly functioning percutaneous breast biopsy team. The nurse, along with the technologist, assists the radiologist in performing automated core biopsy. In addition, and perhaps most important, the nurse must interact effectively with the patient, her family and/or support persons, and her physicians.

The entire biopsy team is responsible for encouraging self-responsibility in the patient and educating her about any procedures she undergoes, about breast cancer, and about breast self-care. Any team member can and should provide what can be lifesaving information about the diagnosis and treatment of breast cancer. Assessing each patient's level of education, expectations, and willingness to learn allows the staff to tailor any information to her level of understanding. As with any procedure, it is important for the health care professional to avoid talking up or talking down to the patient. Useful information can be gathered from general conversation with the patient about her job, family, interests, and previous experiences with breast problems or related issues (1).

PATIENT CONCERNS

The woman who has been referred for an image-guided core biopsy reacts in a variety of ways. Uppermost in her mind is the underlying fear of breast cancer. Even though most breast lesions biopsied are benign, the patient's fear of the possibility of cancer often outweighs her fear of the procedure.

Assessing how the patient is coping with the recommendation for a core biopsy begins immediately when the patient agrees to undergo the procedure. At this time the newness of the terminology and information

can be overwhelming. The patient may also be concerned that her questions will give the appearance of ignorance (2). Although health care personnel usually concentrate on the medical aspects of a procedure, patients often focus more on the outcome of the procedure and its effect on their families than on the procedure itself (3).

A recent study suggested that preoperative anxiety may depend more on a patient's personal coping style than on the specific medical condition (3). Treating each patient as an individual may reduce her anxiety more effectively than relying on preconceived assumptions about why patients are anxious. Weinberger et al. (4) described a simple coping-style model, *repression-sensitization*, which works well for determining the approach to take for patient teaching. *Repression-sensitization* refers to the usual way in which people react to the threatening aspects of a situation. Repressors tend to deny or minimize the anxiety they are experiencing. They may brush off teaching attempts with statements such as, "Let's get on with it," and "I don't really want to know." Women who have repressor traits usually appreciate being told succinctly what they have to know to complete the procedure. The staff can then add short comments throughout the biopsy. If the staff feels rejected by patients with the repressor style, they need to recognize that these patients still need to feel safe and secure. Sometimes a touch, a look, or a kind word helps promote these feelings more than does in-depth conversation.

Sensitizers are more likely to exaggerate their anxiety. They ask many questions, keep the nurse at their sides, and seek lots of information. To avoid delay of the procedure, one can encourage this type of patient to "come with me and I will continue to answer questions as we go along." These women enjoy "chit-chatting" and having the nurse close by during the entire procedure. If the nurse needs to be away for a moment, she should inform the patient and let her know that

J.P. Camp: Radiology Imaging Associates, Breast Diagnostic and Counseling Centre, Englewood, Colorado 80111.

she'll return promptly if possible. To feel safe these patients need to be cared for actively. They appreciate receiving brochures and other information and the offer of a cup of coffee or other beverage when appropriate.

It is fairly common for health care professionals to become annoyed with patients who experience extreme anxiety before a minor procedure such as core biopsy (3). It is important to remember, however, that core breast biopsy is not routine or minor to a patient. The unknown is frightening. Even though the staff may perform several of these procedures a day, the patient undergoes only one. Although the nurses, technologists, and physicians may routinely perform other much more dangerous interventional procedures, most patients cannot compare their experience with the needle biopsy to other procedures. Women who have had surgical biopsy or other surgical procedures generally tolerate needle biopsy much more easily than women who have had no previous invasive procedures. Acknowledging a woman's individuality and treating her with respect and courtesy can help minimize any impatience and intolerance the health care professional may be experiencing. It is important to remember that, when the patient begins to feel safe and comfortable, her tolerance for the procedure will increase, allowing optimal cooperation.

Patient comfort is substantially affected by the physical environment and location of the facility. The Breast Diagnostic and Counseling Centre (BDCC) (Englewood, Colorado) is located in a modern, medical office building surrounded by attractive landscaping. The building is in a technological business complex several miles from the nearest hospital. The location and parking are very accessible, which eliminates the need for patients to hunt for parking or to search for the Breast Centre itself. The decor was planned to nurture female patients. The furnishings and soft colors in the reception area and patient examining rooms could be used comfortably in a home. Soft background music, up-to-date magazines, and decaffeinated coffee and tea are provided.

Most importantly, the entire staff is prepared to assist women through what is sometimes a very emotionally draining procedure. Everyone from the telephone schedulers and receptionists to the health care providers is oriented to listening to and caring for the patients.

A patient recently commented, "I immediately felt safe and important." Contrast this with the experience often found in a large inpatient institution. Patients can feel intimidated by the immense size of some hospital complexes. Patients are directed to various places before they reach their final destination and are often asked the same questions by many different people. Even in smaller hospitals, patients can be shifted from one place and person to another, following signs and

lines to reach their destination. Even extremely competent and efficient hospital staff can come across as aloof and somewhat uncaring because of the environment. A woman visiting a hospital for "just a breast exam" may not be top priority because there are emergency cases and patients with more serious illnesses who take precedence. Many hospitals are beautifully appointed, but somehow the patients do not feel safe and important. A woman with a breast problem generally does not feel sick and does not need the surroundings where sick people reside (i.e., hospitals). If it is necessary to perform core biopsy within a hospital, it is important to give patients a sense of separation from the hospital itself.

REFERRAL

At the BDCC, patient referrals for core biopsy are accepted from primary-care physicians and surgeons. Occasionally, the radiologist interpreting the diagnostic imaging studies will immediately contact the patient's physician to recommend needle core biopsy. The biopsy may then be performed as part of the diagnostic workup at the patient's initial visit or scheduled within a few days. The patient's comfort level is always given top priority in decisions about when and if the biopsy is performed.

Self-referrals initiated by the patient are also accepted at the BDCC. These patients are asked to identify their primary physician and bring along or send all films with their reports and recommendations. If further studies are needed, they are performed at the initial visit. The patient's physician is contacted before proceeding with a core biopsy, and then copies of all reports are sent to the physician.

PATIENT COUNSELING BEFORE BIOPSY

It is extremely important for the nurse or technical staff member to obtain pertinent information about the patient before her biopsy. Typically, this occurs when the referring physician or patient telephones to schedule the biopsy appointment. The information necessary for patient assessment is listed in Appendix A. Information that should be given to the patient when she makes her appointment is listed in Appendix B. Gathering this information and providing instructions to the patient may seem cumbersome but can usually be completed in less than five minutes. A pamphlet describing the procedure is most helpful and can be provided to the patient by the breast center or her referring physician.

After the admission papers are completed, the nurse accompanies the patient and her spouse or support person to a quiet, comfortable, and private office for the informed consent conference (Fig. 1). Here the nurse discusses the biopsy procedure and postbiopsy instructions in detail with the patient and, if the patient chooses, with her spouse or support person. The patient is also informed that her physician will have the results of the biopsy the next day or the next working day if a holiday or weekend intervenes. The patient is asked whether she has further questions and then is asked to repeat her perception of the procedure and on which breast it is to be performed. Sometimes the patient asks for further clarification of the exact breast problem and its location. She may even want to see her mammogram and/or ultrasound films. If she would like to speak with the radiologist, this is also done at this time. The nurse or radiologist then witnesses the signing of the informed consent (5). See Appendix C for possible informed consent content.

It is very important during the informed consent conference to assess the patient's emotional status carefully, to support and reassure her, and to let her know who will be present throughout the procedure. If for any reason she is hesitant about the procedure, this should be communicated to the radiologist, who will then speak with the patient. If the patient requests that the procedure not be performed, the radiologist notifies her physician.

When the informed consent process is completed, the nurse accompanies the patient to the dressing room. The BDCC has an enclosed room with dressing cubicles and individual lockers so the patients maintain a sense of privacy. The patient is instructed to remove her clothing from the waist up and is provided with an attractive cotton gown that ties in front. For a recumbent stereotactic core biopsy, the patient will be lying prone with her head turned to one side and flat on the table. She will be more comfortable without earrings and glasses.

EQUIPMENT

The biopsy tray set-up is minimal. With the exception of the sterile biopsy guide used for stereotactic biopsy, the trays are identical for both stereotactic and ultrasound-guided biopsy. The Mayo stand and sterile tray with the necessary supplies and instruments are shown in Fig. 2 and described in Appendix D.

The BDCC adapted specific policies for sterilization and disinfection, basic aseptic technique, and operating room environmental sanitation from the Recommended Standards and Practices of the Association for Operating Room Nurses (AORN) (6). Nondisposable instruments are autoclaved or soaked in a disinfectant solution containing glutaraldehyde, following the specific directions for use on the container. Sterile thumb forceps and/or sponge sticks are used to hand sterile items like syringes to the radiologist. Universal precautions must also be strictly followed. Hazardous wastes such as syringes, needles, scalpels, and blood-contaminated materials must be disposed of according to standard guidelines after the biopsy (7).

Lidocaine hydrochloride 1%, mixed 10:1 with sodium bicarbonate (50 mOsm/mL), is used to anesthetize the skin and superficial breast tissues. Usually 5 to 10 mL are sufficient. Neutralizing the acidity of the lidocaine with sodium bicarbonate virtually eliminates the stinging sensation when the anesthetic is administered. This is particularly important when performing a stereotactic biopsy because, if a patient flinches from the anesthetic and moves her breast, the coordinates must be recalculated.

Although epinephrine can cause minor skin irritation and occasionally skin necrosis if used as a skin anesthetic, a 1:100,000 mixture of lidocaine hydrochloride 1% and epinephrine can be used to anesthetize deeper regions within the breast. This, of course, requires a longer needle, which is described below. If the patient states that she has an adverse reaction to epinephrine, lidocaine without epinephrine may be used for the entire procedure. If a patient states that she does not react well to procaine lidocaine should still be considered safe to use. If the patient is unsure of a specific drug reaction, it may be best to check with the pharmacist or the patient's physician and to inform the radiologist.

Vasovagal reactions to the image-guided, needle core biopsy performed in the recumbent position are

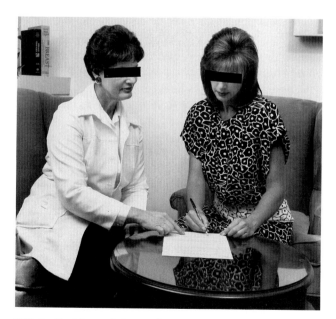

FIG. 1. Prebiopsy informed consent and counseling conference. The patient is counseled about the details of the core-biopsy procedure and then signs the informed consent. This usually takes about ten minutes. (Courtesy of Geoffrey Wheeler.)

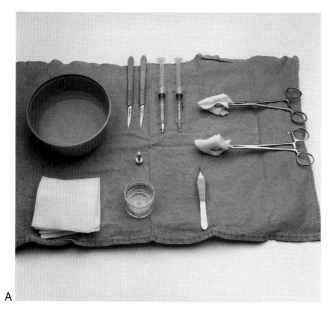
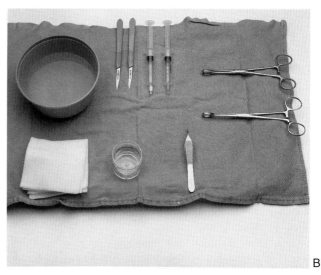

A

B

FIG. 2. A: Sterile tray for stereotactic biopsy. The sterile tray includes two sponge forceps with folded sterile 4 × 4 pads; two 6-mL syringes with the local anesthetic and sodium bicarbonate mixture; two scalpels with #11 blades, one for making the skin nick and one for removing core tissue from the needle; sterile 4 × 4 pads; the needle guide; and a basin with sterile water. **B:** Sterile tray for ultrasound biopsy. The sterile tray includes two sponge forceps, a small thumb forceps, two 6-mL syringes with the local anesthetic and sodium bicarbonate mixture, one scalpel with a #11 blade, sterile 4 × 4 pads, and a basin with sterile water. (Courtesy of Geoffrey Wheeler.)

virtually nonexistent, as are other severe reactions. However, in the unlikely event of an emergency, it is best to be prepared with oxygen, emergency drugs, ammonia nitrate ampules, one-way resuscitation\cardiopulmonary resuscitation (CPR) masks, and an intravenous (IV) setup. Mild vasovagal reactions can usually be controlled with cold cloths to the forehead and back of the neck, while the nurse instructs the patient to breathe slowly and deeply and talks with her. No patient has experienced a severe reaction to the procedure at the BDCC.

An occasional patient would benefit from mild consciousness sedation with benzodiazepines (e.g., Versed) or barbiturates [e.g., methohexital sodium (Brevital)]. Oral sedatives may be taken beforehand, or IV access can be established for IV sedation. Those patients with IV sedation should be monitored for signs of underventilation or apnea throughout the procedure and for approximately 30 minutes after completion. Monitoring includes assessment of heart rate, intermittent blood pressure, respiration rate, continuous pulse oximeter, and level of consciousness. An Ambu bag must be available during the procedure with an appropriate emergency backup system. Patients can also be given an antitussive medication before the biopsy if coughing might be a problem.

The biopsy procedure from the technologist's perspective is described in Chapter 5. The radiologist's perspec-

tive on stereotactic and ultrasound-guided biopsy is described in Chapters 7 and 13, respectively.**

STEREOTACTIC BIOPSY: RECUMBENT POSITION

After the patient has been counseled and has changed into a gown, she is accompanied to the biopsy room by the nurse or technologist and briefly oriented to the equipment. At this time the patient's blood pressure and pulse are taken and recorded while the patient is sitting on the stereotactic biopsy table.

The technologist and the nurse assist the patient in assuming a prone position with her breast through the opening in the table. Patient comfort can be enhanced by placing a pillow under her knee, a paper head towel under her face, and a rolled towel under her contralateral shoulder. A blanket can be provided for warmth (Fig. 9 in Chapter 7).

The patient is usually more cooperative and less anxious when she is made as comfortable as possible before compressing her breast. The nurse can often assist the technologist in placing the breast in compression, especially with posterior lesions and/or small-breasted patients. Explaining to the patient the importance of not moving her breast is critical. The nurse can help the patient remain still by staying close and talking with her. Keeping within the patient's range of sight is important as the patient must not move her head lest she moves her breast in the process. During these first few minutes, while the technologist is obtaining the films and repositioning as necessary, the patient will often "settle in" and relax. The nurse can help by staying close, lightly massaging the patient's neck and shoulders, and being very attuned to what she is communicating, verbally and nonverbally.

When the preliminary films are complete, the nurse or tech preps the portion of the breast exposed in the compression-plate window with povidone-iodine (Betadine) swabs. The nurse or technologist then puts the biopsy assembly on the stereotactic unit. She places the sterile insert into the needle guide and positions the Biopty gun with the sterile 14 gauge needle in its holder. The radiologist becomes actively involved with the biopsy after these steps are completed. The lesion's coordinates are calculated on the computer and transferred to the biopsy-guidance device for needle placement. (See Chapters 5 and 7.)

After the biopsy gun and needle are aligned on the proper trajectory, the radiologist anesthetizes the skin using a 25 gauge, ⅝-inch needle and the deeper breast tissue using a 25 gauge, 1¼-inch needle. The radiologist makes a tiny skin nick with a #11 blade on a disposable scalpel. After the radiologist advances the needle to the computed depth, stereo views are obtained documenting the prefire needle position. The button on the biopsy gun is pushed to obtain tissue, and a final set of postfire stereo views is made. Radiologists at BDCC inform the patient before each click of the biopsy gun so she will not be startled by the sound. After the radiologist backs the needle out of the breast, the core is placed in a sterile specimen cup with saline. Gentleness is crucial in removing the core from the needle. Vigorously swishing the needle in the saline or scraping the core out of the sample notch can damage or fragment the specimen. At least five good quality specimens are obtained. To provide compression and minimize bleeding between passes, the nurse holds a folded sterile 4 × 4 pad with a sterile sponge stick between the needle guide and the patient's breast each time the biopsy needle is withdrawn (Fig. 3). Ten percent formalin is added to the specimen cup to fix the cores before sending them for pathologic examination. In cases with microcalcifications, specimen radiography is performed before fixing to verify the presence of microcalcifications (see Chapter 5).

As soon as the procedure is finished, the compression plate is released. The nurse washes the breast with sterile water to remove the povidone-iodine and any blood, lowers the table, and assists the patient to a sitting position.

The nurse maintains compression at the biopsy site

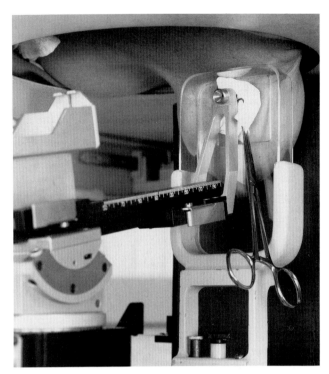

FIG. 3. Pressure to minimize bleeding. After the biopsy needle is withdrawn, the sponge stick with a folded sponge is placed between the needle guide and the patient's breast. (Courtesy of Geoffrey Wheeler.)

with a sterile 4 × 4 pad for five minutes or until bleeding ceases. Bleeding is very slight, but the compression helps to minimize any bruising that may occur over the next 24 hours. A Steristrip is placed over the needle puncture site, pulling the two skin edges together. The nurse applies a small pressure dressing over the biopsy site; the dressing comprises a folded sterile 4 × 4 pad with another sterile 4 × 4 pad placed over it and taped tightly in place (Fig. 4). Usually one long strip and two very short pieces of tape over the 4 × 4 pad provide adequate pressure. Paper or silk tape can be used if the patient is sensitive to Transpore tape. Postprocedure blood pressure and pulse are recorded and are often lower than the prebiopsy vital signs.

The patient is then accompanied to the dressing room by the nurse. Here an ice pack (a 3- × 5-inch resealable plastic bag with small ice cubes) is placed on top of the pressure dressing, inside the patient's brassiere. After dressing, the patient is offered juice, water, or decaffeinated coffee or tea. The nurse gives the patient written biopsy instructions (Appendix E) to reinforce the verbal instructions provided before and during the biopsy. The patient is asked to return on the following day for the nurse to assess her breast postbiopsy. The patient is then free to leave.

During the postbiopsy assessment on the following

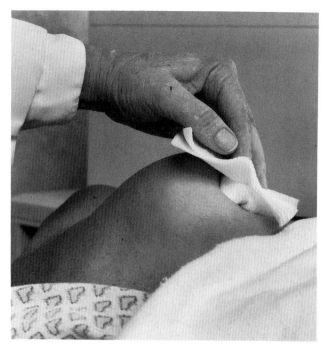

FIG. 4. Pressure dressing. A Steristrip draws the edges of the skin together. Then a pressure dressing is applied to minimize bruising. (Courtesy of Geoffrey Wheeler.)

day, it is important that the nurse appraise the patient's experience with the procedure, answer any questions, and remind the patient that her physician will have the pathology report later in the day. Excessive bruising, tenderness, or evidence of an additional palpable finding can be evaluated with ultrasound and clinical examinations. Bruising and tenderness have been minimal in over 1,000 cases, and significant hematomas have not occurred. If a small hematoma occurs, aspiration can be attempted. When the patient cannot return for clinical follow-up, she is contacted by telephone, and the importance of the recommended follow-up is reinforced.

The pathology department is contacted on the following day, and the report is taken verbally and/or by fax. The referring physician is contacted with the preliminary results either by the nurse or by the radiologist. Unless otherwise directed, the radiologist and breast center staff have the patient discuss the results of her biopsy with her referring physician. Some radiologists and/or the referring physicians may prefer that the radiologist informs the patient of the results.

ULTRASOUND-GUIDED BIOPSY

The prebiopsy procedure for ultrasound-guided core biopsy is nearly identical to that for stereotactic core biopsy. The only difference is that the patient may wear glasses or jewelry as they will not interfere with

the procedure or her comfort. Patient positioning is naturally different because ultrasound-guided biopsy is done in the oblique supine position. The nurse helps the patient remove her arm from the gown on the affected side and lie on her back with her head on a pillow. A second pillow is placed under her knees for comfort, and a blanket is provided for warmth. A wedge is placed under her shoulder on the affected side, and her arm is raised above her head where it rests comfortably on the pillow (Fig. 5).

The nurse preps the patient's breast with two povidone-iodine swabs, starting from the nipple and extending outward in a circular motion well beyond the area of the lesion. The entire breast surrounding the prepped area is draped with three sterile towels on which sterile 4 × 4 pads are placed (Fig. 6). The radiologist can wipe off excess gel and any blood with these 4 × 4 pads. Sterile ultrasound gel is then placed over the breast lesion. Alcohol can also be used as a coupling agent.

Wearing sterile gloves, the radiologist anesthetizes the skin and deeper breast tissue and makes a tiny skin nick, as described under "Stereotactic Biopsy." Holding the transducer in one hand and the needle in the other, the radiologist directs the needle into the breast and toward the lesion using ultrasound guidance. A nonsterile assistant, either the nurse or the technologist, holds the nonsterile Biopty gun to stabilize the handle. When the radiologist has correctly positioned the needle, he or she tells the patient to listen for the click of the biopsy device. The assistant then pushes the button on the biopsy gun. Again, alerting the patient before firing the gun can prevent her from being

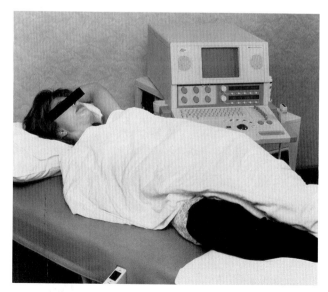

FIG. 5. Patient positioned for ultrasound-guided core biopsy. The patient lies on her back with pillows under her knees and under her head for comfort. A blanket can also be provided for warmth. (Courtesy of Geoffrey Wheeler.)

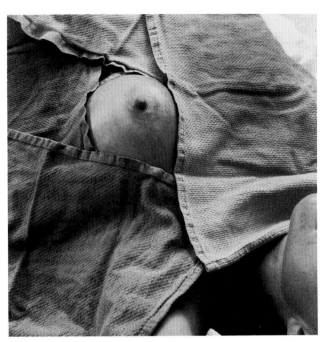

FIG. 6. Breast prepared for ultrasound-guided core biopsy. The entire breast is prepped by swabbing povidone-iodine in a circular fashion from the lesion outward. Sterile towels are draped around the entire breast. (Courtesy of Geoffrey Wheeler.)

startled by the sound. Also, directing the patient's attention to the ultrasound monitor can divert her attention away from the needle entering her breast.

After the needle has been removed from the breast, it is taken out of the gun, and the tissue core is gently placed in sterile saline in the sterile specimen container. The rest of the procedure is the same as that described for stereotactic biopsy.

CONCLUSION

Careful and thorough assessment, education, and counseling by the nurse can make the patient's experience of a core biopsy a positive one. The nurse is in a key position to encourage the patient to take responsibility for her health care and to maintain good breast health. The nurse can also assume many of the patient care responsibilities before, during, and after the biopsy, thus freeing the radiologist to attend to other patients, procedures, or film interpretation.

REFERENCES

1. Bauer-Creamer C, Webber M. Patient teaching strategies for peripheral laser procedures. *Prog Cardiovasc Nurs* 1990;5(2): 50–58.
2. Burkhart LE. The nurse's role as clinical coordinator for the Center for Cranial Base Surgery. *J Neurosci Nurs* 1991;23(1):61–63.
3. Domar AD, Everett LL, Keller MG. Preoperative anxiety: is it a predictable entity? *Anesth Analg* 1989;69:763–767.
4. Weinberger DA, Schwartz GE, Davidson JR. Low anxious, high anxious and depressive coping styles: psychometric patterns and behavioral physiological responses to stress. *J Abnorm Psychol* 1979;88:369–380.
5. Glass E. Informed consent: the nurse's role. *Cancer Nurs News* 1990;8(1):3.
6. *AORN recommended standards and practices.* Denver: American Association of Operating Room Nurses; 1992.
7. *Occupational exposure to blood borne pathogens; final rule.* Federal Register Part II. Washington, DC: Occupational Safety and Health Administration, Department of Labor; December 6, 1991.

APPENDIX A

Information Obtained from Patient\Physician When Scheduled

1. *Identifying information:* Name, birth date, phone numbers: home/work
2. *Referring physician:* If patient schedules the appointment herself, it is important to know if she has discussed this procedure with the person she states is her referring physician.
3. *Breast imaging information:*
   Previous mammography and/or ultrasonography
   Location of the lesion
   Visualization on mammography and/or ultrasound
   Palpability and by whom
4. *Location of films* with instructions to the patient to bring her films and the reports with her if applicable
5. *Medical history:* Cardiac problems, diabetes, allergies (Also, it is helpful to know whether the patient has limitations that would cause problems lying prone on the stereotactic table.)
6. *Medications:* Anticoagulants: Current prothrombin time (PT) and partial thromboplastin time (PTT) studies should be performed.
   Aspirin: Is she taking daily doses of aspirin, aspirin derivatives, or other drugs related to clotting deficiencies?
   Prophylactic antibiotics: Does she need prophylactic antibiotic therapy for mitral valve prolapse, artificial heart valves, etc.
7. *Allergies:* Allergic reactions to local anesthesia/ epinephrine

APPENDIX B

Prebiopsy Instructions

1. Come ten minutes before your appointment to complete the necessary paperwork.
2. If possible, avoid aspirin or aspirin derivatives for 48 hours or preferably one week before the biopsy.
3. It is unnecessary to restrict eating and drinking before the biopsy.
4. Makeup, deodorant, and other hygienic measures will not interfere with the biopsy.
5. The total appointment including pre- and postbiopsy counseling and paperwork will take 1 to 1½ hours.
6. You may return to your work or other activities on the day of your biopsy if they do not involve heavy lifting or strenuous athletic activities. On

the following day all activities should be well tolerated.

APPENDIX C

Informed Consent

1. Date
2. Patient's name
3. Description of the procedure (in lay terms)
4. Statement of the reason for the procedure
5. Reference to a few general complications and/or risks
6. Anesthesia
7. Reference to the specific\serious complications of the procedure
8. Alternatives to the procedure
9. Patient's signature after a short paragraph stating that an explanation has been given, that the form has been read and understood, that the patient's questions have been answered, and that the patient wishes to proceed.
10. Witness to signature

APPENDIX D

Tray Set-up

Sterile Tray

Mayo stand covered with sterile towel
Basin with sterile water
8 sterile 4 × 4 pads
1 small thumb forceps
One 6-mL syringe with a 25 gauge ⅝-inch needle with local anesthetic (without epinephrine)
One 6-mL syringe with a 25 gauge 1¼-inch needle with local anesthetic (containing epinephrine)
1 disposable scalpel with a #11 blade
2 sponge sticks
empty for ultrasound biopsy
with sterile 4 × 4 pad for stereotactic biopsy
Needle guide (stereotactic biopsy only)

Other Supplies (Not on Tray)

Nonsterile gloves for assistant(s)
Sterile gloves for radiologist
Two sterile povidone-iodine swabs (packaged)
Sterile specimen container with ¼-inch sterile saline

Biopty gun and sterile 14 gauge 16-cm biopsy needle
Steristrips
Tape
3 × 5 resealable plastic bag with ice

APPENDIX E

Care After a Needle Core Biopsy

1. Place an ice pack inside your bra on top of the dressing until bedtime.
2. Remove the pressure dressing the next morning after the biopsy. Do not shower or bathe until you remove the pressure dressing.
3. Remove the Steristrip two days after the biopsy. You may bathe your breast carefully with the Steristrip in place. Be careful not to loosen it.
4. You may have mild discomfort, and you may have a small amount of bruising where the needle entered the skin.
5. If you need medication for discomfort, take acetaminophen products such as Tylenol or ibuprofen products such as Advil, Nuprin, Motrin, etc. Do not take aspirin for 24 to 48 hours.
6. Do not participate in strenuous activities for 24 hours—tennis, aerobics, weight lifting, skiing, etc.
7. Watch for excessive bleeding, pain, or fever. If any of these occur, contact the Breast Centre or your doctor.
8. Please return to the Breast Centre the next day to have the biopsy site checked by the nurse. This will take only a few minutes. If your biopsy is done on a Friday, please call on Monday for follow-up.
9. Your doctor will receive a verbal report within 24 hours unless this would be on a weekend, in which case your doctor will receive the report on Monday. Please contact him/her between 2 and 5 p.m.
10. Please make an appointment at the Breast Centre in _____ for a _____ exam of the _____ breast to establish a new base line examination and to recheck the area where the biopsy was performed.

Percutaneous Breast Biopsy, edited by
Steve H. Parker and William E. Jobe.
Raven Press, Ltd., New York © 1993.

CHAPTER 5

The Technologist's Role

Gina Simon

The technologist's primary responsibilities in both stereotactic and ultrasound-guided core biopsy are operating the imaging equipment and monitoring quality assurance. (For specific pitfalls to avoid in operating stereotactic equipment, see Chapter 6.) The technologist also positions the patient and consults with the radiologist about selecting the most appropriate imaging technique and approach to each lesion.

A good team approach involves coordinating the duties of the radiologist, nurse, and technologist in all aspects of the biopsy and ensures that the patient receives the best possible care. Although the nurse counsels the patient before the biopsy, it is equally important for the technologist to make the patient feel at ease during the procedure. The technologist and nurse share the responsibility for making the patient as physically comfortable as possible, allowing her to relax and cooperate during the procedure. Everyone involved in the biopsy must be sympathetic and responsive to the patient's emotional state. At the BDCC the patient is never left alone before, during, or after the procedure, and each member of the biopsy team is capable of reassuring and educating her.

STEREOTACTIC BIOPSY

Stereotactic biopsy from the radiologist's point of view is described in Chapter 7. Figure 1 is a diagram of the Fischer Mammotest, to which reference is made in this chapter and in Chapters 4, 6, and 7. Appendix A contains Mammotest features and technique recommendations.

G. Simon: Radiology Imaging Associates, Breast Diagnostic and Counseling Centre, Englewood, Colorado 80111.

Calibration Check

The technologist checks the machine calibration every morning to ensure pinpoint accuracy when performing the actual biopsy (Appendix B). A phantom consisting of a plastic block with four embedded BBs is used to calibrate the machine (Fig. 2A). The phantom is placed in the compression device so that all four points are within the opening in the compression paddle (Fig. 2B). A stereo film is taken and taped securely to the digitizer for programming. Coordinates for each BB are taken (Fig. 2C). After the punction instrument and needle are placed on the tube arm, the micrometer is set for the horizontal, vertical, and depth coordinates of the first BB. The needle is advanced against the phantom. The tip should touch the BB and be dead center (Fig. 2D). This process is repeated for each simulated lesion. The deepest BB is the most sensitive to error because, the greater the distance the needle travels, the more chance of deflection. This is referred to as *distance error*.

Patient Positioning

For a stereotactic core biopsy using a dedicated, recumbent stereotactic unit, the patient lies prone with the indicated breast through the table aperture (Fig. 9 in Chapter 7). The patient is in a slight left or right anterior oblique position with the affected breast forward and the opposite shoulder elevated. A headrest is not recommended because of the stress it puts on the patient's neck. Instead, a towel placed beneath the patient's face is usually most comfortable. A small wedge sponge can be used for patients who prefer a headrest. A rolled towel placed under the elevated shoulder provides additional neck support, allowing the patient to relax against the cushion. A pillow under the knee on the same side as the elevated shoulder can

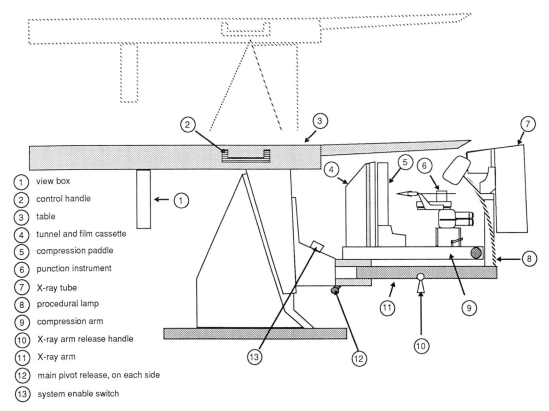

1 view box
2 control handle
3 table
4 tunnel and film cassette
5 compression paddle
6 punction instrument
7 X-ray tube
8 procedural lamp
9 compression arm
10 X-ray arm release handle
11 X-ray arm
12 main pivot release, on each side
13 system enable switch

FIG. 1. Side view of the Mammotest table detailing its components. (Courtesy of Fischer Imaging Corporation, Denver, Colorado.)

reduce stress on the patient's back. Making the patient as comfortable as possible to minimize any chance of movement is extremely important. At this point, raising the table to its highest level allows the radiologist, nurse, and technologist the most comfortable working position.

Repositioning, restereoing, and redigitizing is required if the patient moves at any point during the biopsy. For monitoring of patient movement after initial positioning, the upper corners of the biopsy window can be marked on the breast with a black felt-tip pen.

Preliminary Views

After the patient is as comfortable as possible on the table, the technologist moves the table top until the desired area of the breast is centered within the compression-paddle window and resting against the cassette holder (Fig. 3). The procedure requires a fair amount of compression; however, it need not be as vigorous as a regular mammogram. The technologist takes a straight scout film to verify that the lesion is seen in the compression plate aperture (Fig. 13 in Chapter 7). After gaining some experience using the equipment, the technologist usually can place the lesion within the window on the first attempt.

Next, preliminary stereotactic views are obtained (Fig. 14 in Chapter 7). Stereo images taken at opposing $+15°$ and $-15°$ (30° apart) provide three-dimensional localization. The technologist places a cassette in the holder, pushes it to the extreme left, and rotates the x-ray tube to the $+15°$ détente position for the first stereo exposure (Fig. 4). For the second exposure, the technologist pushes the same film to the extreme right and rotates the tube to the $-15°$ détente position. Suggested manual techniques are outlined in Appendix C.

The breast can be biopsied with the tube in the craniocaudal, the 45° or 90° mediolateral, or the lateral-medial position. The tube angle that provides the shortest needle path from the skin to the lesion is preferred. The technologist measures the skin to lesion distances on craniocaudal, mediolateral or 90° lateral views of the original mammogram (Fig. 5). In conjunction with the radiologist, the technologist then decides which tube angle offers the shortest route and adjusts the tube and the patient's breast accordingly. When the distance is equal on both the craniocaudal and the mediolateral view, the view in which the lesion is best visualized or in which the needle traverses the least amount of fibrous tissue is best.

Although most areas are easily positioned within the compression device, difficult cases, particularly lesions close to the chest wall, may need special atten-

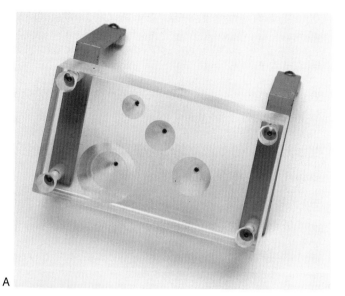

A

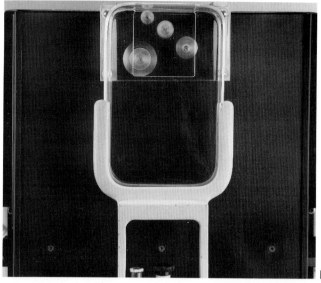

B

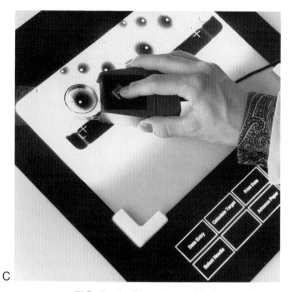

C

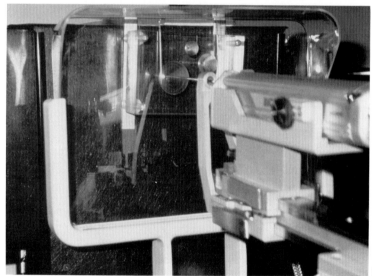

D

FIG. 2. A: Phantom with four embedded BBs for calibration of the Mammotest unit. **B:** Phantom placed in the compression device with all four points within the compression-paddle opening. **C:** Coordinates for each BB are entered on the digitizer. (**A, B, C** are courtesy of Geoffrey Wheeler.) **D:** Needle advanced against the phantom with the needle tip dead center on the BB.

tion even from experienced technologists. When faced with a more difficult case, persistence pays off. First, the technologist must know how to select the proper compression paddle (Fig. 6). The standard paddle works well when lesions are in the midbreast. However, with calcifications and/or lesions close to the chest wall (Fig. 7A), the smaller adjustable paddle is a better choice. Adjusting this paddle to extend higher into the aperture allows better visualization of the posterior breast tissue (Fig. 8). Dropping the affected shoulder slightly into the table aperture will also bring more breast tissue into the field of view.

The patient's shoulder may obscure the area of interest on one or both of the stereo views when it is dropped into the table aperture to visualize very posterior or axillary lesions (Fig. 7B,C). This happens because of the 15° angle of the tube arm. Occasionally, tape can be used to lift skin folds out of the field of view, making it possible to visualize a very posterior lesion that would otherwise be obscured. It may be necessary to wear a lead apron while holding the shoulder and axillary skin folds out of the field of view.

The smaller paddle also works well with anterior lesions, especially those near the nipple, where spot

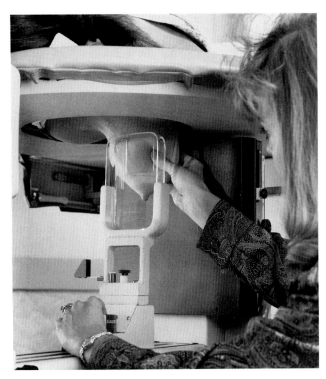

FIG. 3. Table top is moved until the desired area of the breast is centered within the compression-paddle window. (Courtesy of Geoffrey Wheeler.)

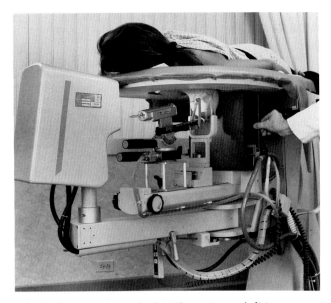

FIG. 4. Cassette is pushed to the extreme left to accommodate +15° rotation of the tube for the first stereo exposure. (Courtesy of Geoffrey Wheeler.)

compression is necessary. Lesions in the lower aspect of the breast, especially the 6 o'clock position, require selecting this paddle for spot compression as well (Figs. 4 to 6 in Chapter 7).

When one is sampling a lesion at the 6 o'clock position, the caudal-cranial position would offer the shortest route to the lesion. This position is not an option with the Mammotest unit (Fischer Imaging Corporation, Denver, Colorado) but is possible with the LORAD unit (LORAD Medical Systems, Danbury, Connecticut). With the Mammotest, the mediolateral or lateral-medial position provides the next shortest route. After the breast is compressed in the lateral position, the needle does not travel significantly farther than it would if the lesion were approached caudal-cranially (Fig. 9). Lesions at the 6 o'clock position requiring biopsy are quite unusual.

In some cases, areas of fibroglandular asymmetry seen on the initial mammogram will not be as apparent on stereotactic mammograms. The smaller compression paddle allows more localized compression than does standard mammography and may demonstrate that the asymmetry is merely a function of compression (i.e., superimposition of fibroglandular tissue). When fibroglandular asymmetry resolves on the stereotactic views, the radiologist may recommend mammographic follow-up rather than biopsy.

The dedicated stereotactic unit has three diaphragms: (a) the larger diaphragm for scout filming, (b) the standard stereo diaphragm, and (c) the smaller T-stereo diaphragm (Fig. 10). In most cases the standard diaphragm is used for stereo imaging. When x-raying an extremely dense or large breast, excessive scatter radiation may overexpose one of the reference cross hairs (Fig. 11). The T-diaphragm reduces the scatter radiation, providing the stereo images with better resolution which accentuates very fine microcalcifications or subtle lesions. The T-diaphragm also shields the reference cross hairs from overexposure and maintains their visibility (Fig. 12). The T-diaphragm does, however, reduce the field of view in comparison to the standard diaphragm. Since tube angulation projects the lesion slightly to one side compared to the opposite stereo view, sometimes the suspicious area cannot be seen on one of the stereo views (Fig. 13). Therefore, positioning the area of interest directly in the center of the window on the original scout is critical in these cases (Fig. 14).

Biopsy Procedures

After the scout and preliminary stereotactic views have been obtained, the remainder of the procedure generally takes 20 to 30 minutes. With an experienced team assisting the biopsy, the radiologist need only be

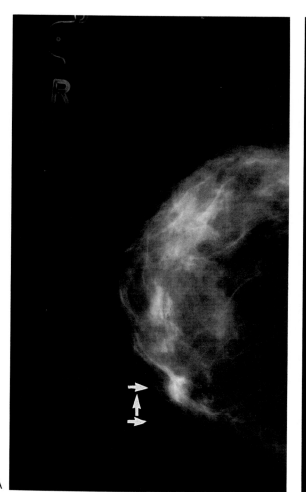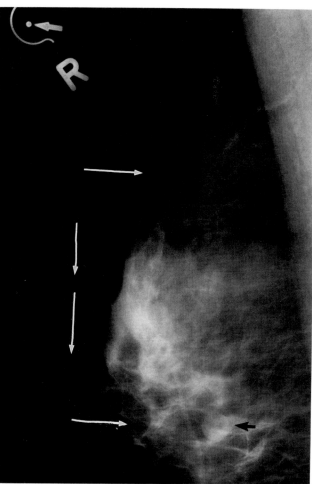

A   B

FIG. 5. Skin-to-lesion distances (*vertical arrows*) are measured on the craniocaudal (**A**) and medio-lateral (**B**) views of the original mammogram. In this case, the mediolateral view is chosen because it provides the shortest path to the lesion (*black arrows*).

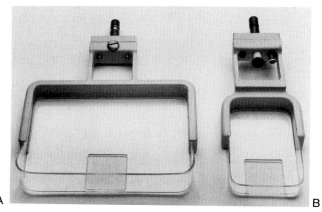

A   B

FIG. 6. A: Standard compression paddle (*left*) used for larger breasts and in localizing lesions in the midbreast. **B:** Smaller adjustable compression paddle (*right*) used in all other cases. (Courtesy of Geoffrey Wheeler.)

present after the technologist has developed the preliminary stereotactic film and placed it on the digitizer. The radiologist then programs the digitizer to determine the coordinates of the lesion, and the technologist or radiologist dials these numbers into the main unit. Automatic alignment devices that eliminate the need to dial in coordinates are also available (Fig. 1 in Chapter 14). The radiologist advances the needle to the desired depth, and the technologist makes two stereo exposures. Taking stereo exposures before and after firing the biopsy gun verifies lesion stability and accurate needle placement.

Processing these films as quickly as possible reduces the patient's time in compression. It is critical that the processor be conveniently located close to the biopsy room. A rotating door makes the darkroom accessible while other films are being developed. Other technologists can help expedite the processing by allowing the biopsy technologist to develop films first. At the BDCC

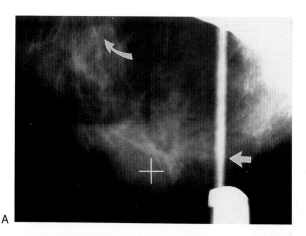
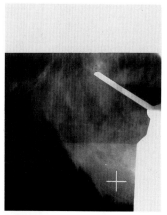
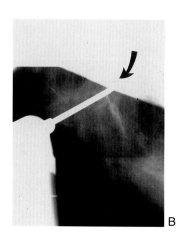

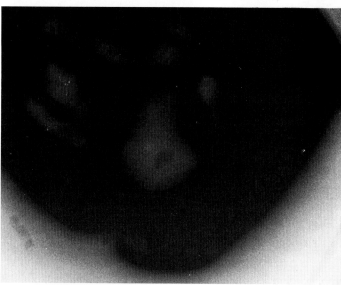

FIG. 7. A: Very posterior microcalcifications (*curved arrow*) requiring the use of the smaller adjustable compression paddle (*arrow*), which pulls more breast tissue into the field of view. **B:** This extremely difficult case required dropping the patient's shoulder (*arrow*) on the affected side into the table aperture. Because of the tube angulation, the calcifications (*arrow*) were difficult to see on the right stereo view. Lifting the skin folds with tape made these calcifications visible. **C:** Persistence paid off in this difficult case. The specimen radiograph verified that calcium was present in the cores.

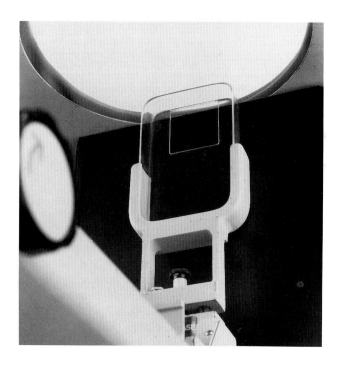

FIG. 8. Small adjustable compression paddle extending higher into the aperture for better visualization of posterior breast tissue. Even though approximately ¼ inch of the film is not exposed because of the table, more breast tissue is pulled into the field of view. (Courtesy of Geoffrey Wheeler.)

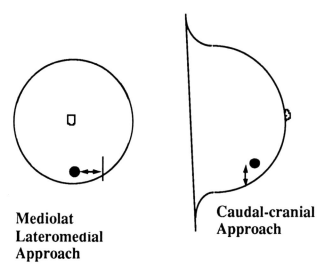

Mediolat
Lateromedial
Approach

Caudal-cranial
Approach

FIG. 9. Diagram demonstrating the distance the needle travels after the breast is compressed in the lateral position for a 6 o'clock lesion. The needle does not travel much farther than if approached caudal-cranially.

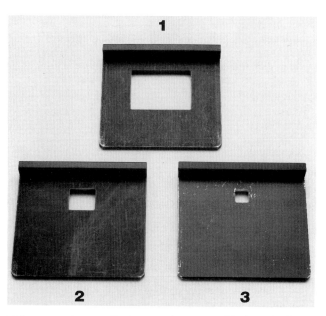

FIG. 10. 1: Large diaphragm for scout filming. **2:** Standard stereo diaphragm. **3:** Smaller T-stereo diaphragm. (Courtesy of Geoffrey Wheeler.)

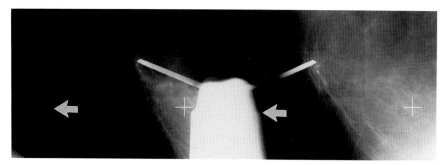

FIG. 11. With the standard stereo diaphragm, scatter radiation overexposed the left reference cross hair (*arrows*).

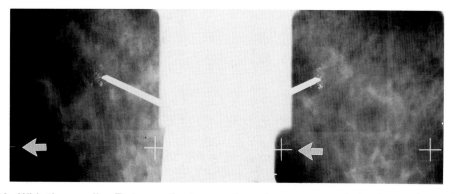

FIG. 12. With the smaller T-stereo diaphragm, the reference cross hairs (*arrows*) are shielded from overexposure.

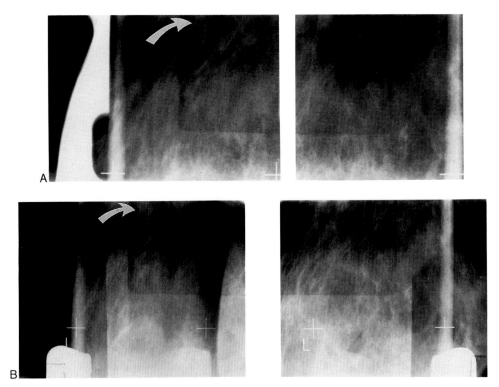

FIG. 13. T-stereo diaphragm (**A**) reduces field of view when compared to the standard stereo diaphragm (**B**). The +15° rotation of the tube causes the lesion in both figures to be projected into the left-hand corner (*arrows*) of the compression-paddle opening.

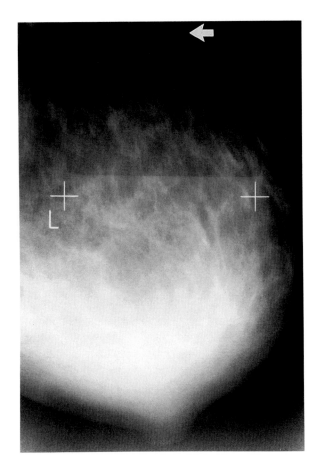

FIG. 14. It is important to position the lesion (*arrow*) as close to the center of the window as possible when scout filming. This will ensure that the angulation does not project the lesion out of the window on the stereo views when the small T-diaphragm is used.

expediting biopsies is important enough that there is an office policy giving the biopsy technologist first priority in the darkroom. Charged coupled devices (CCDs), which produce near real-time digitized images, eliminate the need for immediate film developing (Fig. 2 in Chapter 14).

After the radiologist has verified proper needle placement by reviewing the pre- and postfire images (Fig. 15), additional cores can be obtained. In most cases no further films are necessary, but on occasion the radiologist may need a final postfire film after minor readjustment of the coordinates.

After the final core is taken, the patient is released from compression. While the nurse holds pressure at the biopsy site, the technologist can prepare the specimens. The specimens are fixed with 10% formalin and sent to the pathologist as soon as possible.

When microcalcifications are biopsied, a specimen radiograph can verify that calcium is present in the cores (Fig. 30B in Chapter 7). For best results this is accomplished by carefully pouring the specimens and a small amount of the accompanying physiologic saline into the lid of the specimen container. A 5-mL syringe can be used to draw off the excess saline so the specimens can be carefully situated for a magnification view. This view should be closely collimated using maximum magnification capability and a technique of 25 mA, 0.1-mm focal spot, and 6 to 8 mAs with a maximum of 23 kV. (See Appendix C for other technique recommendations). This will provide optimum visual-ization of the calcifications. Since it is extremely important to fix the specimens as soon as possible, the specimen radiograph should be taken immediately after the biopsy.

In busy practices the technologist can expedite the schedule by preparing the films and paperwork for the next patient while the nurse sees the previous patient out. The technologist can then prepare the biopsy room for the next patient, who is being counseled by the nurse.

Quality assurance is described in detail in Chapter 6.

ULTRASOUND-GUIDED BIOPSY

Patient Positioning

Both types of biopsy (stereotactic and ultrasound) can be performed on the Mammotest table. For ultrasound cases a pillow is simply placed over the opening in the table to support the patient's head.

For an ultrasound-guided biopsy, the patient lies in an oblique supine position with a wedge sponge under the affected side (see figure 6 in Chapter 4). When the right breast is biopsied, she lies in a left posterior oblique position, and vice versa for the left breast. Placing the ipsilateral arm above her head evenly distributes the breast tissue.

Preliminary Preparations

Most ultrasound equipment uses image-processing controls that are sometimes displayed in the data field alongside the ultrasound image (Fig. 16). The technologist works with the service representative during installation to preset these controls for optimum visualization of breast tissue. A brief description of these controls follows:

The *gray scale* (contrast) controls the shades of gray assigned to the ultrasound image. Visualizing solid masses and tumors within a background of fatty tissue requires an image with considerable contrast.

Persistence (frame averaging) can enhance tissue differentiation to allow visualization of subtle tissue changes. Maximum tissue differentiation is required for breast imaging. However, too much persistence can blur the image.

Edge enhancement enhances the lesion boundaries and controls the smoothness of the image. Medium edge enhancement is useful for accentuating boundaries with 7.5 mHz transducers in small-parts scanning.

Compression (dynamic range) represents the range of gray scale shades assigned to different levels of sound intensity. The widest dynamic range produces the lowest contrast image, and the narrowest dynamic range produces the highest contrast image.

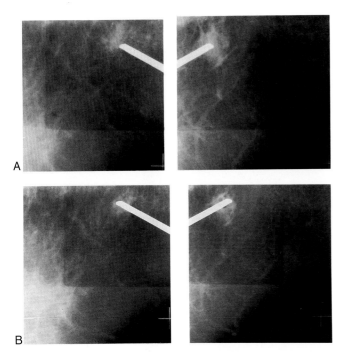

FIG. 15. A: Prefire images document proper needle alignment. **B:** Postfire views document proper needle alignment.

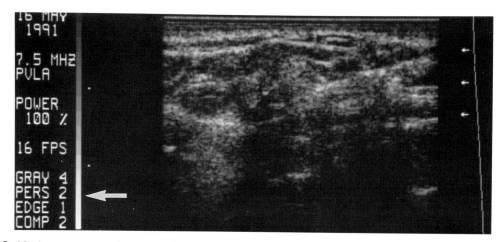

FIG. 16. Image-processing controls (*arrow*) displayed in the data field to the side of the ultrasound image on the 5200 Acoustic Imaging System (Acoustic Imaging, Phoenix, Arizona). (Courtesy of Geoffrey Wheeler.)

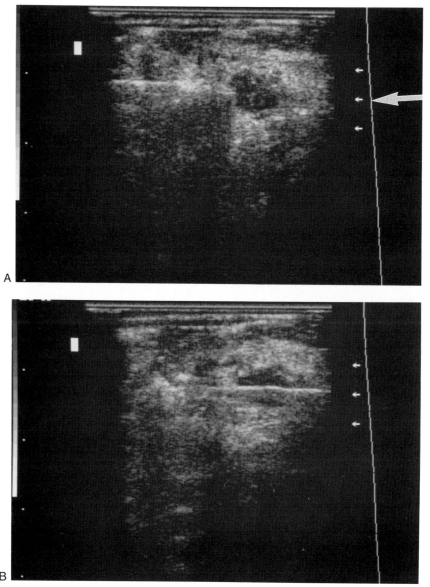

FIG. 17. A: Prefire ultrasound image of the needle in line with the lesion. **B:** Postfire ultrasound image of the needle coursing through the lesion.

The *output power* is measured in decibels (db) and varies the amount of sound energy sent into the body. Settings range from 0% (off) to 100% (maximum).

Time gain compensation (TGC) allows an increase, decrease, or overall amplification of echoes at various depths. It is usually displayed on the monitor as a sloping line near the image. The technologist adjusts the TGC until the desired image is obtained.

The *focal zone control* focuses the ultrasound beam. The technologist adjusts the focal zone(s) to the desired scan depth, covering the lesion being biopsied (see *arrow* in Fig. 17A). Adding too many focal zones slows the frame rate and can create a "windshield-wiper" effect deterring from real-time visualization.

A 7.5 mHz linear array transducer is recommended. The technologist soaks the transducer in glutaraldehyde for a minimum of 15 minutes before the procedure. The technologist must ensure that no fluid enters the transducer or the cable entry point, since complete immersion in fluid can permanently damage the transducer. Soaking just below the level of the cord will prevent accidental leakage into the transducer.

Once the patient is prepped and the ultrasound machine settings are correctly adjusted, the radiologist localizes the lesion and needle under the transducer. The radiologist then takes core samples (see under "Stereotactic Biopsy"), documenting accurate target-ing with pre- and postfire images. It is important for the technologist to obtain good images of the needle both in line with the lesion (prefire) and through the lesion (postfire) (Fig. 17).

As with the stereotactic biopsy, the technologist can expedite the schedule by preparing the specimens and developing the films while the nurse attends to the patient after the biopsy. At the BDCC one technologist assists both stereotactic and ultrasound-guided biopsies, so the technologist must rearrange and prepare the room between patients regardless of the imaging method chosen.

Ultrasound-guided biopsy from the radiologist's point of view is described in Chapter 13.

Conclusion

It is important that the technologist be well versed in mammography, the principles of stereotaxis, ultrasound's application in the breast, and quality assurance of both ultrasound and mammography equipment. It is helpful for the technologist to be knowledgeable about film review so he or she can assist the radiologist in selecting the appropriate approach to a given lesion. Finally, combining the efforts of the nurse, radiologist, and technologist ensures the best possible care for the patient.

APPENDIX A

Mammotest Features and Technique Recommendations

The Mammotest unit has a source to image distance (SID) of 68 cm for high-resolution images.

A rotating 10° molybdenum target provides adequate radiation output for short exposures.

A large focal spot size (FSS) of 0.4 mm is used to accommodate the 100- and 125-mA station.

Kilovolt selections are available in 0.5-kV increments up to 20 to 39 kV.

Milliampere-second selections are available in varying increments from 1 to 750 mAs.

Automatic exposure control (AEC) density selections are available in 11 steps, with a 12.5% change per step.

Phototiming/AEC may be used for initial scouting but is not recommended for stereo imaging. The angle of the tube (+15° and −15° degrees) inhibits proper utilization of the photocell.

For optimum contrast images use less than 30 kV, if possible.

For increased contrast on fatty breast tissue, decrease 1 to 2 kV from normal.

For more adequate penetration with a shorter exposure time on dense breast tissue, increase 1 to 2 kV from normal.

APPENDIX B

Calibration Procedure

The calibration procedure is as follows:

1. Warm up the tube.
   a. Turn on the power switch to the generator and computer.
   b. Turn off the phototimer.
   c. Set the mAs at 120 at 27 kV.
   d. Make 3 exposures—wait approximately 15 seconds—repeat twice.
2. Zero the micrometer.
   a. Place the punction instrument on the tube arm.
   b. Turn the dials (both horizontal and vertical) to 00.00. Make sure that the mechanical zeroes and the zeroes on the micrometer agree. If they do not agree, call for service before proceeding.
3. Calibrate the computer.
   a. Place the Mammotest phantom on the stereo tunnel, making sure that all four points are within the opening in the compression paddle.
   b. Compress the phantom to hold it in place. It is a good idea to tape it down to ensure lack of movement.
   c. Take stereo film—always take the first exposure with the tube on the right side of the table.
4. Develop the film.
5. Place the film in holders on the computer. The "L" should always be on your left. Tape the film down to ensure that there is no movement.
6. Using the mouse on the computer, select the appropriate needle size. A 16-cm needle is recommended.
7. Move the data entry and take coordinates for each simulated tumor.
8. Place the punction instrument on the tube arm.
9. Set the micrometer for the horizontal, vertical, and depth measurements for the first simulated lesion.
10. Place the appropriate needle guide in the needle-guide holder. For the needle guide to accommodate the needle, it must be the same gauge. A 14 gauge needle is recommended, so a 14 gauge needle guide must be used.
11. Load the needle into the Biopty gun, cock the gun, and engage the safety.
12. Gently place the Biopty gun on the punction instrument securely within the sled.
13. Advance the needle-guide holder against the phantom.
14. Advance the needle holder to the correct depth. Do not forcefully advance the needle against the phantom because it might bend the needle tip.
15. The tip of the needle should touch the BB in the phantom and must be dead center.
16. Repeat the same process for each simulated lesion.
17. If the needle is not dead center on the BB and the needle is not bent, redo the procedure in Step above. If it continues to be off, do not perform the biopsy. Call the service engineer to correct the problem.

APPENDIX C

Manual Non-Bucky Screen Techniques

Breast	Compression (cm)	kV	mAs
Small	1–3	28	80–125
Medium	3–6	29	125–175
Large	6–9	30	175–250
Specimen		23	6–8

The film, chemicals, and processor used to accommodate techniques are listed below:

Kodak MRE-1 Min-R Film
Kodak RP X-omat
Developer and replenisher
Fixer and replenisher
Kodak X-omat
270 RA Processor
Extended 3 minute processing

The Mammotest system accepts Kodak Min-R cassettes and screens.

Percutaneous Breast Biopsy, edited by
Steve H. Parker and William E. Jobe.
Raven Press, Ltd., New York © 1993.

CHAPTER 6

Principles of Stereotactic Mammography and Quality Assurance

R. Edward Hendrick and Steve H. Parker

Stereoscopic acquisition and viewing of breast radiographs dates back to 1930, when Stafford L. Warren, a radiologist at Strong Memorial Hospital, Rochester, New York, reported using a screen-film stereoscopic technique for *in vivo* mammography (1). Stereoscopic acquisition and viewing of mammograms and other mammographic procedures fell into disfavor with the demonstration that radiation could induce mutations and breast cancer in laboratory animals (2) and with the recognition of the relatively high radiation doses involved in early mammography (3).

After marked reduction of radiation doses was achieved for mammography, the stereotactic approach was reevaluated. In the last decade, stereotactic localization has been used clinically to guide the placement of wires to mark suspicious breast lesions in preparation for surgical biopsy. More recently, stereotactic localization has been used to guide fine-needle aspiration and large gauge core biopsies of the breast (4–10).

Large-core biopsy and fine-needle aspiration biopsy are discussed in Chapters 7 and 9, respectively.

THE PRINCIPLES OF STEREOTACTIC LOCALIZATION

Stereotactic localization uses two planar radiographic views acquired at different x-ray source positions to determine the location of radiographically visible objects in three spatial dimensions. Assuming that the patient is placed in the prone position with her breast dependent (Fig. 3 in Chapter 5), the three spatial

dimensions of a breast lesion are x (horizontal position), y (vertical position), and z (distance into the breast measured from the back breast support) (Fig. 1). The two acquired planar radiographs differ only in the horizontal position and direction of the x-ray source. Figure 2 is a top view schematic of the stereotactic system with the breast under compression. Stereotactic views are acquired with the x-ray beams directed at $+15°$ and $-15°$ relative to a line perpendicular to the image receptor. Other angles may be used; these are the particular stereotactic angles used on the Mammotest stereotactic system (Fischer Imaging, Denver, Colorado). Using a collimated x-ray beam, a single screen-film cassette is sufficient for the acquisition of both views. The cassette is shifted horizontally to the right for acquisition of the $+15°$ view and to the left for the $-15°$ view, so that images of the two views do not overlap. An example of a stereotactic pair of scout images of a 1-cm breast lesion is shown in Fig. 3. A pair of " + sign" cross-hair reference markers in each image are radiopaque markers located in the plane of the back breast support.

The x (horizontal) location of the lesion, when approached from the 0° or perpendicular ray (the approximate line of approach of the biopsy needle), is the average of the x locations of the lesion in the two views. The y (vertical) location of the lesion is the same in both views, since the only changes from one view to the other are the horizontal shifts of the x-ray tube and the cassette; there is no vertical shifting from one view to the other. The z location (or depth) of the lesion is determined by the amount of parallax shift of the lesion from one view to the other, as shown schematically by Fig. 4. If the two views are obtained without moving the image receptor and x_{ls} is the parallax shift of the lesion on the image receptor from the $+15°$ view to

R.E. Hendrick: Department of Radiology, University of Colorado Health Sciences Center, Denver, Colorado 80262.

S.H. Parker: Radiology Imaging Associates, Breast Diagnostic and Counseling Centre, Englewood, Colorado 80111.

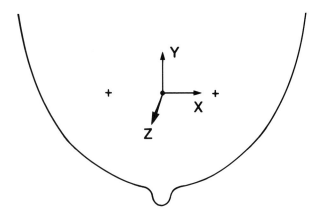

FIG. 1. The three-dimensional coordinate system used to define the location of breast lesions. The x and y coordinates are parallel to the plane of the image receptor. The z axis is perpendicular to the plane of the image receptor, with the $+z$ direction pointing back toward the x-ray source (when oriented at 0°).

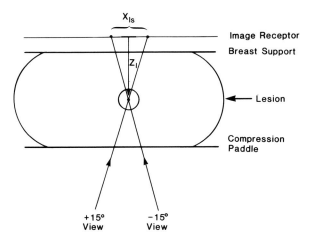

FIG. 4. A schematic of the parallax shift of a lesion on a fixed image receptor (x_{ls}) and its geometric relationship to the distance of the lesion from the image receptor (z_l).

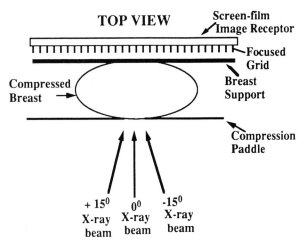

FIG. 2. A schematic top view of the stereotactic localization system.

the $-15°$ view, by simple geometry the distance of the lesion from the image receptor (z_l) is

$$z_l = \frac{x_{ls}}{2\tan(15°)} = 1.866 \cdot x_{ls} \qquad [1]$$

In Fig. 3, the image receptor has been moved between the $+15°$ and $-15°$ views so that the two images are not superimposed. In this case the parallax shift of the lesion is measured relative to the two cross hairs that appear in each image. The lesion projects slightly farther to the right relative to the cross hairs in the $+15°$ view (the image on the left) than in the $-15°$ view. The shift in lesion position from one stereotactic view to the other, measured relative to the radiopaque cross hairs in each image, is $x_0 = x_{ls} - x_{ms}$, where x_{ls} (lesion shift) is the shift in position of the center of the lesion from one image to another and x_{ms} (marker shift) is the shift in position of a cross hair from one image

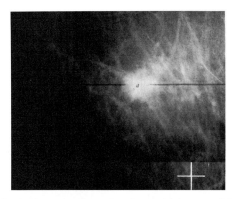
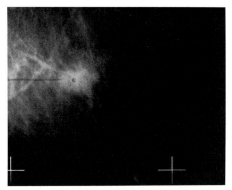

FIG. 3. A stereotactic pair of scout images obtained on a patient with a 1-cm lesion. The $+15°$ view is on the left, and the $-15°$ view is on the right. A pencil point has been added at the center of each lesion to aid in entry of lesion coordinates. A pencil line has been drawn through the two center points to verify that the line through the centers is parallel to the line through the "+" reference markers in the two films.

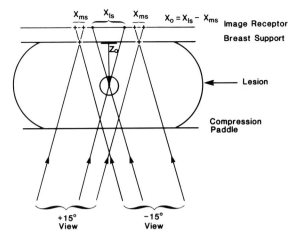

FIG. 5. A schematic of the relative shift of a lesion on an image receptor, $x_0 = x_{ls} - x_{ms}$, and its geometric relationship to the distance of the lesion from the plane of the reference markers (z_0).

to another (see Fig. 5). Thus, x_0 is the shift of the lesion relative to the markers from the $+15°$ view to the $-15°$ view. The distance of the lesion from the back breast support, z_0, is then given by

$$z_0 = \frac{x_0}{2\tan(15°)} = 1.866 \cdot x_0 \qquad [2]$$

Equation 2 applies whether the image receptor is moved between acquisition of the two stereotactic views or not. The equation says that, if the lesion does not shift relative to the cross hairs between the two views ($x_0 = 0$), then the lesion is at the same depth as the back breast support ($z_0 = 0$). The shift of the lesion relative to the cross hairs indicates the perpendicular distance of the lesion from the back breast support (z_0). This, in turn, indicates how far to insert the biopsy needle to place the tip of the needle at the center of the lesion.

Thus, all three coordinates of the breast lesion (x, y, and z) can be determined from the two stereotactic views. If different angular settings are used to acquire the stereotactic views (e.g., $+20°$ and $-20°$), then that different angle should be used in Eqs. 1 and 2 (instead of 15°) to determine the z location of the lesion.

THE METHOD OF STEREOTACTIC LOCALIZATION AND BIOPSY

The nurse's, technologist's, and radiologist's points of view regarding core biopsy are described in Chapters 4, 5, and 7, respectively.

The specific steps in stereotactically guided needle biopsy of breast lesions are listed below.

1. The breast is compressed with the lesion positioned within the window of the compression paddle (Fig. 3 in Chapter 5).

2. A 0° scout film is acquired and processed to confirm that the lesion is centered within the window of the compression paddle (Fig. 6).
3. A +15° scout film is acquired with the x-ray source positioned 15° to the left of perpendicular and the cassette pushed to the right.
4. With the same cassette, a −15° scout film is acquired with the x-ray source positioned 15° to the right of perpendicular and the cassette pushed to the left.
5. The scout film is processed (Fig. 3).
6. The scout film is placed on the digitization table, and the positions of the two cross hairs and the center(s) of the lesion(s) are entered from both the +15° and the −15° views (Fig. 15 in Chapter 7).
7. The computer calculates and prints the horizontal, vertical, and depth coordinates of the center of the lesion.
8. A sterilized needle is placed in the biopsy gun, and the gun is cocked and then mounted on the punction arm, which consists of the biopsy gun holder and the alignment mechanism (Fig. 7). A sterilized needle guide is also placed on the punction arm.
9. The specified horizontal and vertical coordinates are entered on the micrometer dials of the punction device (Fig. 18 in Chapter 7), and the biopsy gun is advanced so that the biopsy needle is at the surface of the breast (Fig. 12 in Chapter 7).
10. A small amount of local anesthetic is given at the location of needle entry to the breast, and a small incision is made at the point of entry of the biopsy needle.
11. The needle is inserted to the specified depth coordinate (Fig. 8) to position the tip of the biopsy needle at the center of the lesion.

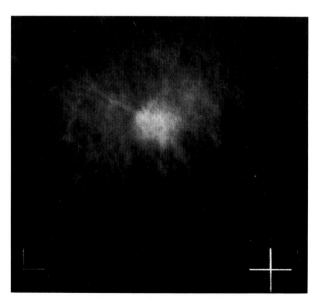

FIG. 6. A 0° scout film confirming that the lesion is within the window of the front compression paddle.

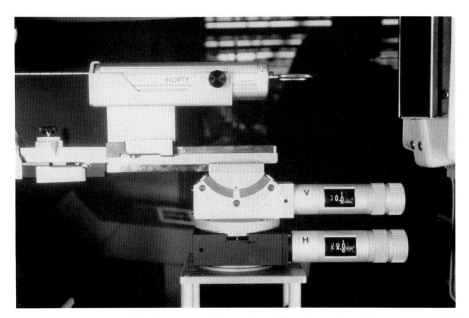

FIG. 7. The biopsy gun, sterilized core needle, and sterilized needle guide are mounted on the punction arm, ready for needle insertion.

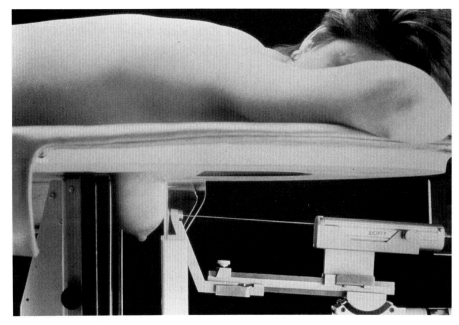

FIG. 8. The core needle is inserted to the specified depth.

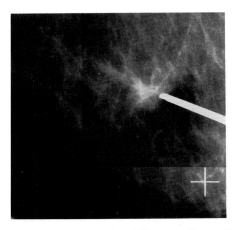
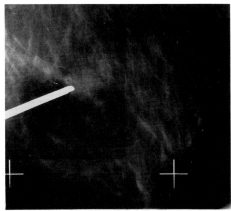

FIG. 9. Prefire +15° and −15° scout films. The tip of the needle should be at the center of the lesion on both views.

12. Prefire +15° and −15° views are acquired on a single cassette and processed to verify that the tip of the biopsy needle is located at the center of the lesion on both views (Fig. 9).
13. The needle is withdrawn 5 mm, and the biopsy gun is fired.
14. Postfire +15° and −15° views are acquired on a single cassette and processed to verify that sampling has occurred through the lesion (Fig. 10). (Steps 12, 13, and 14 are described in detail below.)
15. At least four additional samples are acquired at slightly different horizontal and vertical locations through the lesion.

THE VERIFICATION OF ACCURATE TARGETING AND SAMPLING

The biopsy gun fires a specially designed needle consisting of two separately moving parts: an inner needle with a biopsy slot and a covering sheath (Fig. 11). When the biopsy gun is fired, the inner needle ad-vances first to penetrate the breast lesion with minimal deflection. The 14 gauge core needle has an inner needle with a solid 4-mm tip followed by a 17-mm slot to capture the sampled tissue. The remainder of the inner needle is solid. The thin covering sheath is fired next to cut the sampled tissue from the breast; the sampled tissue is retained in the slot of the inner needle. The entire needle (inner needle and covering sheath) is then withdrawn, and the sampled tissue is removed from the needle for examination by the pathologist.

Verification that the tip of the needle is at the center of the lesion requires that the tip of the needle project symmetrically over the center of the lesion in *both* the +15° and −15° prefire views, as shown schematically in Fig. 12. It is not sufficient to have the tip of the needle project over the center of the lesion in one view, as in Fig. 13. In fact, seeing some space between the tip of the needle and the margin of the lesion in either of the prefire images indicates with certainty that the lesion will be missed. The lesion may also be missed if the needle appears symmetrically short of the lesion (Fig. 14) or beyond the lesion (Fig. 15) in both views.

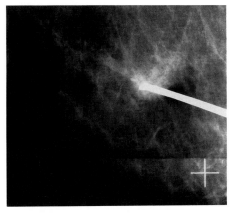
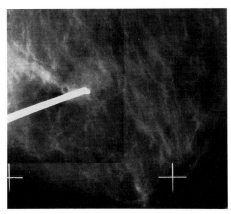

FIG. 10. Postfire +15° and −15° scout films. The tip of the needle should be beyond the center of the lesion on both views.

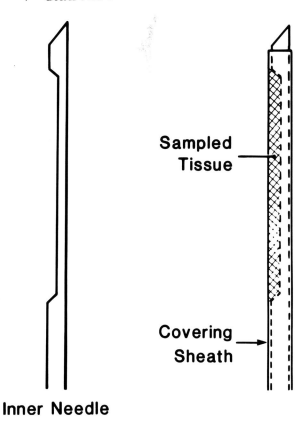

Inner Needle

FIG. 11. Schematic of the two-part 14 gauge cutting needle.

The stroke length is the distance the needle advances during firing. For 14 gauge needle core biopsies using the long-throw biopsy gun, the stroke length is 23 mm. The needle is backed up approximately 5 mm (from the position where the tip of the needle is at the center

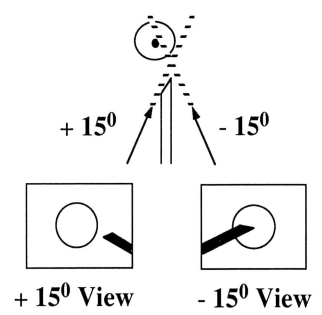

FIG. 13. If the tip of the needle is outside the lesion in either the +15° or the −15° view, the needle has not been properly localized.

of the lesion) before firing to ensure sampling through the entire lesion. This is illustrated in Fig. 16, assuming biopsy of a 1-cm-diameter lesion. Firing the needle from its position with the tip of the needle at the center of the lesion samples only the last 3 mm of the lesion. By backing the needle up 5 mm, the needle samples through most of the lesion, even if the 1-cm lesion moves forward during sampling by as much as 1 cm. Newer needles have different length characteristics and the amount of pullback therefore varies.

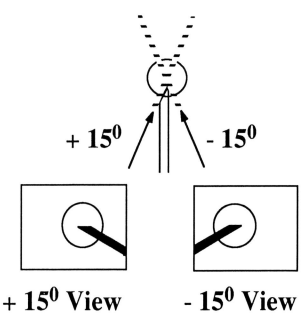

FIG. 12. The location of the needle in +15° and −15° views when the needle is at the center of the lesion.

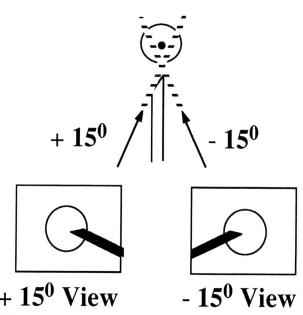

FIG. 14. Appearance of the needle in +15° and −15° views when the needle is symmetrically localized short of the lesion.

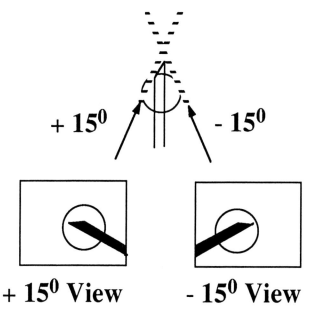

FIG. 15. Appearance of the needle in +15° and −15° views when the needle is symmetrically localized beyond the center of the lesion. This is typical of the desired appearance of the postfire images.

The extent of sampling can be verified by carefully examining the postfire images. However, the dimensions of both lesion and needle have been altered by two factors: a geometric magnification factor (the lesion and needle are geometrically magnified by the divergent x-ray beam imaging objects not in contact with the image receptor) and an angular magnification factor (due to the angulation of the x-ray beam relative to the image receptor). The geometric magnification factor is $m_g = z_{tot}/(z_{tot} - z_l)$, where z_{tot} is the source-to-image receptor distance and z_l is the distance of the lesion from the image receptor. For a lesion at the back breast

support, $z_l = 1.0$ cm and $m_g = 1.02$; for a lesion 6 cm in front of the back breast support, $z_l = 7$ cm and $m_g = 1.11$ (z_{tot} is 68 cm, and the back breast support is 1 cm from the image receptor on the Mammotest unit). The angular magnification factor for the lesion is $m_a = 1/\cos(15°) = 1.035$. The dimensions of the lesion in the image are increased by an overall magnification factor $m_{lesion} = m_g \cdot m_a = m_g/\cos(15°)$, which ranges from 1.06 for a lesion at the back breast support to 1.15 for a lesion 6 cm in front of the back breast support. To correct for this magnification, the lesion size in the image should be divided by m_{lesion} to determine the true lesion size.

The length of the biopsy needle in the pre- and postfire images is foreshortened by the glancing (15°) angle between the needle and the x-ray beam, while being geometrically magnified, just as the lesion. Assuming that the needle approaches the lesion at 0° horizontal and vertical angles (no left-right or up-down angulation), the needle length in the image is an overall factor of $m_{needle} = m_g \cdot \tan(15°) = 0.268 \cdot m_g$ of the actual needle length, where m_g is the geometric magnification factor given above. With m_g ranging from 1.02 to 1.11, the needle length magnification factor will range from 0.273 to 0.298 (the needle length is minified in the image). The actual needle length is the needle length measured in the +15° or −15° views divided by this magnification factor (or multiplied by a factor of 3.663 to 3.356, respectively). Hence, the needle length is foreshortened in the image, whereas the lesion is slightly magnified in the image.

ERRORS IN LOCALIZATION

Several types of errors can occur in stereotactic localizations. They range from errors that can damage

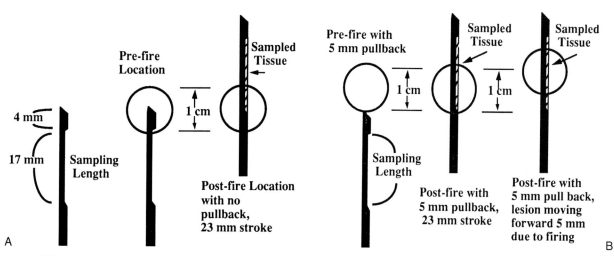

FIG. 16. The 14 gauge sampling needle beside a 1-cm lesion. **A:** If the needle is fired from its position with the tip of the needle at the center of the lesion, only the upper few millimeters of the lesion will be sampled. **B:** If the needle is backed up 5 mm and then fired, sampling is through most of the lesion, even if the lesion moves forward during firing.

the punction device or breast support to errors that can produce incorrect positioning of the biopsy needle, leading to missed lesions.

Operator errors that can damage the equipment include applying excessive pressure to the punction arm. This can occur by leaning on the punction arm or by trying to cock the biopsy gun while it is mounted to the punction arm. The biopsy gun should be cocked only when it is detached from the punction device. The result of excessive pressure can be a bent punction arm or stripped gears on the punction device, both leading to incorrect localizations and requiring repair of the punction device.

A second operator error that can damage the equipment is firing the needle into the back breast support. The long-throw biopsy gun has a stroke length of 23 mm. If the prefire location of the needle tip is within 23 mm of the back breast support, when fired the needle will strike the back breast support, damaging the breast support, possibly bending or breaking the needle, bending the needle guide, and damaging the biopsy gun and punction arm. The stroke margin is defined as the distance of the needle tip from the back breast support *after the biopsy gun has been fired,* assuming that the needle was fired from the center of the lesion without being withdrawn. A positive stroke margin means that the needle tip will remain short of the back breast support after firing. A negative stroke margin means that the needle tip will strike the back breast support if the needle is not withdrawn before firing. When a negative stroke margin occurs, the needle should be withdrawn far enough to ensure that the breast support is not struck when the gun is fired. An extra margin of 3 mm should be added to the length of the negative stroke margin to determine how far the needle should be withdrawn before firing. For example, if a stroke margin of -6 mm is reported, then the needle should be withdrawn 9 mm before firing. This should ensure that the needle tip will remain 3 mm away from the breast support after firing.

At the top of the list of errors that can lead to missed lesions is patient motion. Prone positioning of the patient minimizes patient motion, but any motion occurring between the $+15°$ and $-15°$ scout films or between the two scout films and core sampling can lead to a missed lesion. Breast motion can also occur if the breast is positioned with excessive tension, causing it to retract during the localization procedure even though compression is firm and the patient does not move. This was the cause of a breast cancer close to the chest wall being missed by stereotactic core biopsy (10). Patient motion or breast retraction may be identified on the prefire images by the tip of the needle being away from the center of the lesion on one or both prefire views.

Other sources of error that will yield inaccurate localizations are listed below.

1. Lesion movement within the breast during core biopsy, most commonly occurring with fibroadenomas and small clusters of calcifications
2. The use of two different radiographically visible lesions or calcification groups on the two stereo scout views in the belief that they represent a single lesion
3. Movement of the film on the digitization table during entry of the lesion or cross hair coordinates
4. The presence of stray magnetic fields or ferromagnetic objects (e.g., refrigerator magnets or ferromagnetic jewelry) on or near the digitization table during coordinate entry
5. Entering of the wrong coordinates on the horizontal and vertical punction device micrometer dials
6. Advancement of an uncocked biopsy gun into the breast
7. Moving of the biopsy gun to the wrong depth coordinate along the punction arm
8. Failure to ensure that the front edge of the biopsy gun is flush with the front of the gun holder during use
9. Slipping of the biopsy gun backward as the gun and needle are being moved forward to insert the needle to the proper depth in the breast; the biopsy gun must be clamped tightly to ensure that slipping does not occur.
10. Entering of the wrong needle or needle dimensions into the computer
11. Bending or deflection of the needle during insertion; placing the needle guide close to the front surface of the breast will minimize needle bending.
12. Excessive temperature changes between calibration and use of the stereotactic equipment; the room should be kept at a constant temperature to within a few degrees Fahrenheit.

All of these errors should show up by the needle tip being inaccurately positioned (i.e., not at the center of the lesion) in the prefire images. If the lesion is missed in the prefire images, the source of error should be determined by checking the entered coordinates, checking that the biopsy gun is cocked and properly positioned, and checking that the needle is not deflected. If none of these conditions is the source of localization error, the needle should be withdrawn, a $0°$ calibration check performed, and the prefire films used as the new scout films to enter the coordinates of the lesion for repositioning of the biopsy needle.

A misestimation of the center of the lesion in *one* of the two stereo scout views leads to an even greater misestimation of the *depth* of the center of the lesion. From Eq. 2, an error Δx in the location of the lesion center in *one view* leads to an error in the *z*-location of the center of the lesion of

$$\Delta z = \frac{\Delta x}{2\tan(15°)} = 1.87\cdot(\Delta x) \qquad [3]$$

If the center of the lesion is misestimated in *both views*, the error in the determination of lesion depth can range from zero (when the center of the lesion is misestimated by the same distance *in the same direction* in the two views) to $3.73\cdot(\Delta x)$ (when the center of the lesion is misestimated by a distance Δx *in opposite directions* in the two views). This possible magnification of errors points to the need to locate the center of the lesion accurately in both scout views.

Other sources of error that might occur seem not to be a serious problem with operation by trained, experienced physicians and technologists. When the errors listed above are avoided, localizations should be accurate to within ±1 mm along all three axes.

QUALITY CONTROL PRACTICES

Quality control practices for conventional screen-film mammography units are fully described in the *American College of Radiology Mammography Quality Control Manuals* (11). Those same quality control practices are essential for stereotactic mammography units. It is imperative that image quality be as good on the stereotactic unit as it is on the conventional mammography unit so that lesions detected by mammography can be visualized, located, and sampled by stereotactic methods. Therefore, the same tests recommended for conventional screen-film mammography should be followed for stereotactic mammography, including both technologist and physicist quality control (QC) tests performed at least at the recommended minimum frequencies (Appendix A). The phantom image quality test, using the same phantom as on the conventional mammography unit, should be performed at least monthly, and more frequently at first, to ensure that image quality during stereotactic localization is at least as good as image quality in conventional mammography.

In addition, two quality control tests unique to stereotactic equipment should be performed before patient use. The first test, to be performed before each new patient, is to check alignment of the horizontal and vertical settings of the punction device. This is done by dialing in 0.00° on both the horizontal and the vertical micrometer dials and then making sure that the reference marks on the device match up with the fixed zero reference marks on the body of the punction instrument (Fig. 7). Similar checks should be performed at +5° and −5° on both horizontal and vertical axes.

The second quality control test that is crucial to perform at least daily before patient use of the stereotactic system is the localization calibration phantom test. Each stereotactic system is provided with a localization phantom (Fig. 2A in Chapter 5) that consists of four radiographically visible markers at four different depths in an acrylic base. In the calibration test, the phantom is mounted on the breast support so that the markers are within the window of the compression paddle. The localization protocol described above (short of firing the biopsy gun) is performed for each of the four markers. When the biopsy needle is positioned at the coordinates determined from the scout film, the needle tip should just touch each marker in the phantom. Any deviation from precise localization should be visible to the operator. Failure to localize the tip of the needle accurately on any marker is an indication of system or operator failure. No patient should be examined using the stereotactic system until the source of failure is determined and corrected.

CONCLUSION

Even as further technical developments and innovations are in progress (see Chapter 14), it seems that stereotactic localization and core biopsy of breast lesions offer great promise. When properly performed, stereotactic core biopsies have the potential to replace surgical biopsy of most breast lesions, reducing the time, cost, and trauma to the patient. This in turn offers the potential of treating breast cancer at earlier stages in women screened by mammography with cancer confirmed by stereotactic needle-guided biopsy, ultimately reducing mortality from breast cancer.

ACKNOWLEDGMENTS

We thank Ms. Meg Thams of Fischer Imaging, Denver, Colorado, for providing some of the photographs used in this chapter.

REFERENCES

1. Warren SL. Roentgenologic study of the breast. *AJR Am J Roentgenol* 1930;24:113–124.
2. Furth J, Furth OB. Neoplastic diseases occurring among mice subjected to general irradiation with x-rays: I. Incidence and types of neoplasms. *Am J Cancer* 1936;28:54–65.
3. Upton A, Beebe G, Brown J, Quimby E, Shellabarger C. Report of NCI ad hoc working group on the risks associated with mammography in mass screening for the detection of breast cancer. *J Natl Cancer Inst* 1977;59:813.
4. Kimme-Smith C. New and future developments in screen-film mammography techniques. *Radiol Clin North Am* 1992;30(1):55–66.
5. Jackson VP. The status of mammographically guided fine needle

aspiration biopsy of nonpalpable breast lesions. *Radiol Clin North Am* 1992;30(1):155–166.

6. Grant CS, Goellner JR, Welch JS, et al. Fine-needle aspiration of the breast. *Mayo Clin Proc* 1986;61:377.

7. Lofgren M, Andersson I, Lindholm K. Ster   ne-needle aspiration for cytologic diagnosis of nonpa   lesions. *AJR Am J Roentgenol* 1990;154:1191–11ᶜ

8. Parker SH, Lovin JD, Jobe WE, et al. Ste   biopsy with a biopsy gun. *Radiology* 1990;176:ℸ

9. Lovin JD, Parker SH, Jobe WE, Leuthke JM, Hopper KD. Stereotactic percutaneous breast core biopsy: technical adaptation and initial experience. *Breast Dis* 1990;3:135–143.

10. Parker SH, Lovin JD, Jobe WE, Burke BJ, Hopper KD, Yakes WF. Nonpalpable breast lesions: stereotactic automated large-core biopsies. *Radiology* 1991;180:403–407.

11. Hendrick RE, Bassett LW, Dodd GD, et. al. *American College of Radiology Mammography Quality Control Manuals.* Reston, VA: American College of Radiology; 1992.

APPENDIX A

Quality Control Tests Listed in the ACR Quality Control Manuals for Conventional Mammography Units (11)

Technologist's Tests	Frequency	Medical Physicist's Tests (All Tests To Be Conducted at Least Annually and After Major Equipment Changes)
Darkroom cleanliness	Daily	Cassette holder assembly evaluation
Processor quality control	Daily	Collimation assessment
Screen cleanliness	Weekly	Focal spot size measurement
View boxes and viewing conditions	Weekly	kVp accuracy/reproducibility
Phantom images	Monthly	Beam quality assessment (Half-value Layer measurement)
Visual checklist	Monthly	Automatic exposure control (AEC) system performance assessment
Repeat analysis	Quarterly	
Analysis of fixer retention in film	Quarterly	Uniformity of screen
Darkroom fog	Semiannually	Breast entrance exposure and average glandular dose measurement
Screen-film contact	Semiannually	Phantom image quality evaluation
Compression	Semiannually	Artifact evaluation

Percutaneous Breast Biopsy, edited by
Steve H. Parker and William E. Jobe.
Raven Press, Ltd., New York © 1993.

CHAPTER 7

Stereotactic Large-Core Breast Biopsy

Steve H. Parker

Pinpointing breast lesions within 1 to 2 mm with stereotactic technique is an extremely important development in mammography. Improved imaging technology, however, represents only half of the ingredients necessary for successful percutaneous breast biopsy. Automated biopsy devices and large (14 gauge) core needles, essential for adequate sampling, compose the other half. Successful stereotactic biopsy can be assured only when both of these components function properly.

The first attempts to combine stereotactic mammography and biopsy guns were made with "add-on" stereotactic units and short-excursion, 18 gauge core needles (1). Initial experiences with add-on units were disappointing (1), although some investigators later reported success with them (2–4) (see Chapter 8). Breast specimens obtained with 18 gauge needles were not entirely satisfactory either. Likewise, short-excursion automated biopsy devices were found to be inferior to the long-excursion variety (1,5,6). The eventual marriage of dedicated recumbent stereotactic mammography, automated long-excursion biopsy guns, and 14 gauge needles produced a percutaneous biopsy as accurate as surgical biopsy (7,8).

To appreciate the full benefit of percutaneous core biopsy, one must understand the drawbacks of surgical biopsy. Surgical breast biopsy has a documented "miss rate" of 2% to 9% (9) (Fig. 1) and is costly for the patient and third-party payers. In addition, the physical and psychologic trauma associated with surgical breast biopsy is much greater than that with core biopsy (Fig. 2). Stereotactic biopsies have a similar or lower miss rate and can be performed for one-quarter to one-half the cost of surgical biopsies without creating subsequent mammographic pseudolesions.

Percutaneous breast biopsy with "add-on" mammog-raphy units, with fine-needles, and with ultrasound is covered in Chapters 8, 9, and 13, respectively.

PATIENT SELECTION

Patients selected for percutaneous large-core biopsy include virtually all of those who would be recommended for surgical biopsy. These include patients who have such highly suspicious mammographic findings as stellate lesions or "casting" ductal calcifications and such moderately suspicious lesions as irregular nodular densities or calcifications in lobular distributions. Less suspicious mammographic findings (e.g., well-defined nodules, asymmetries, or vague calcifications) can be biopsied when patient and/or physician concern is high.

In spite of the low cancer yield in "probably benign" lesions, some cancers are still found. Low-suspicion lesions are usually biopsied at the BDCC in patients whose physicians support their desire to confirm benign lesions rather than to endure the uncertainty of short-interval mammographic follow-up.

Any suspicious lesions noted ultrasonographically, regardless of whether or not they are seen mammographically, can be biopsied with ultrasound guidance. Percutaneous automated large-core biopsy is also especially useful in patients with lesions seen well in only one mammographic projection, multiple lesions in one or both breasts, or questionable lesions in postbiopsy patients and in patients who are nursing.

The only patients not routinely biopsied at the BDCC are those suspected of having a radial scar because the higher number of proliferative processes associated with radial scar increases the risk of developing a cancer. The mammographic appearance of a radial scar can mask what would otherwise be recognized as a suspicious mammographic abnormality in its vicinity. Also, pathologists frequently need the entire lesion to

S.H. Parker: Radiology Imaging Associates, Breast Diagnostic and Counseling Centre, Englewood, Colorado 80111.

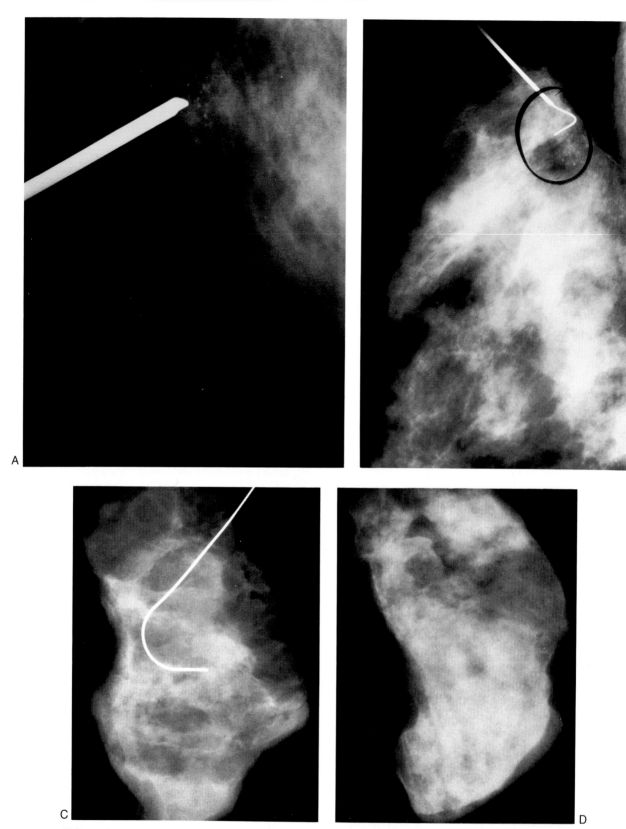

FIG. 1. Surgical "miss." **A:** Stereotactic view of the prefire position of the needle with clustered calcifications at the tip of the needle. The diagnosis from the stereotactic biopsy was DCIS. **B:** Localization of calcifications for lumpectomy with the hook wire in a reasonably good location. **C:** Specimen radiograph of the initial surgical specimen showing the wire without any calcifications in the specimen. **D:** Specimen radiograph of the second specimen from the same patient, again showing no calcifications. The procedure was terminated after the second unsuccessful excision. The area of calcifications and/or DCIS remained on the subsequent mammogram. The patient ultimately underwent successful repeat excision of the DCIS.

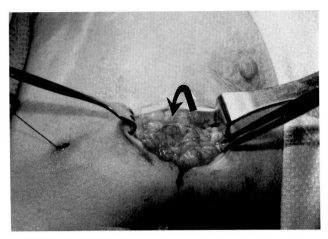

FIG. 2. Open surgical biopsy. The surgeon has intersected the path of the localization wire (*arrow*). (From Parker and Jobe, Ref. 9a, with permission.)

make a definitive diagnosis of radial scar, and core biopsy may not contain enough of the lesion to make the precise diagnosis. However, some argue that, because a radial scar is a benign lesion, the exact histologic diagnosis of radial scar is not necessary and it does not need to be surgically excised (Fred Burbank, *personal communication*). They reason that a needle-core diagnosis of fibrosclerosis from a mammographically stellate lesion suspected of being a radial scar is adequate reassurance.

Some physicians believe that clustered microcalcifications may also not be as well suited to stereotactic

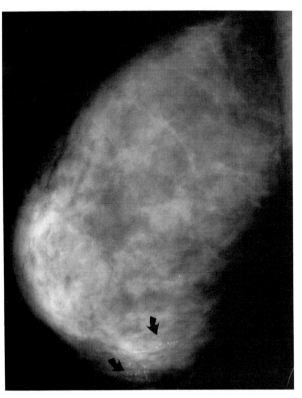

FIG. 4. Dense casting/branching calcifications. Mediolateral mammogram showing areas of calcifications (*arrows*).

breast biopsy as are solid lesions (6). Most, mistakenly, do not differentiate between the different types of calcifications. Since breast microcalcifications are heterogeneous entities, they should be divided into at least two large general categories: less distinct granular calcifications located within the lobule (Fig. 3) and more dense, "broken needle tip" or "crushed stone" calcifi-

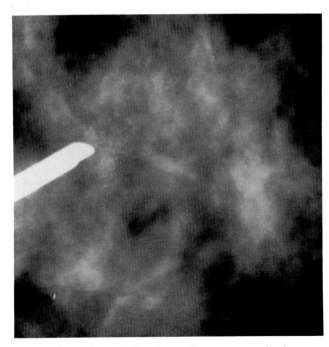

FIG. 3. Granular calcifications. The core needle is seen in the prefire position. The core diagnosis was cribriform DCIS.

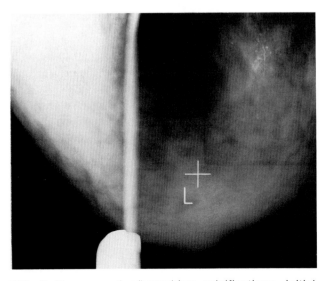

FIG. 5. Dense casting/branching calcifications. Initial scout view.

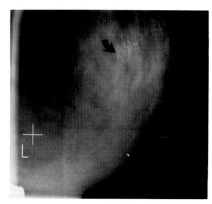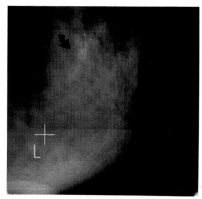

FIG. 6. Dense casting/branching calcifications. Stereotactic views demonstrating the area to be targeted (*arrows*). The histologic diagnosis was high-nuclear-grade DCIS.

cations within the lobule or cast along the duct(s) (10–12) (Fig. 4).

Of the two, core biopsy of granular or "cotton ball" microcalcifications is more controversial because these calcifications, regarded as markers for diffuse disease (either benign or malignant) somewhere in the breast segment, are not necessarily inherently associated with the responsible lesion (11). Theoretically, however, extensive core sampling (i.e., vigorously canvassing such an area of calcifications with ten or more 1.5-cm-long, 14 gauge cores) should be as effective as minimal excisional biopsy (Fig. 3).

Core biopsy of casting and "broken needle tip" or "crushed stone" calcifications is less controversial. Unlike granular calcifications, which are associated with nonnecrotic processes, these calcifications are caused by necrosis (11). Thus, casting calcifications are inherently associated with the disease process causing them, and biopsy of these calcifications should always lead to the correct diagnosis (Figs. 5 and 6).

PATIENT WORKUP

Naturally, all patients who are eventually selected for percutaneous breast biopsy first have screening and/or diagnostic mammograms. Patients who are screened elsewhere and then referred to the BDCC for diagnostic mammography are worked up thoroughly at their initial visit to the BDCC and are almost always biopsied the same day. The same is true for patients referred directly for diagnostic evaluation of a clinical finding.

Prebiopsy workup may include magnification mammography, extra mammographic views (e.g., exaggerated craniocaudal), breast ultrasound, and/or ductography (Fig. 7). Often ultrasound can further characterize mammographic nodules. The ultrasonographic finding of a simple cyst means the biopsy can be canceled. Ductography can identify suspected intraductal papillomas or carcinomas that may not be immediately visi-

ble on mammography or ultrasound (Fig. 8A). Once located with ductography, these lesions can be targeted with mammography or ultrasound for biopsy (Fig. 8B). Mammographic magnification views are especially useful in cases of microcalcifications. These views may demonstrate that the calcifications are more numerous than suspected or are associated with an otherwise undetected soft tissue density. Areas of the cluster associated with a mass and/or subsets of the most suspicious calcifications can be more heavily targeted than was originally planned based on the standard mammogram. Additional views that define a lesion's location more precisely let the radiologist choose the appropriate path to that specific location.

Occasionally, magnification or additional views reveal that a lesion is truly of low suspicion and need not be biopsied. In this case both the patient and her doctor are advised of the mammographic findings. Although canceling the biopsy is recommended to the patient and the patient's physician, frequently a tremendous amount of momentum already exists to per-

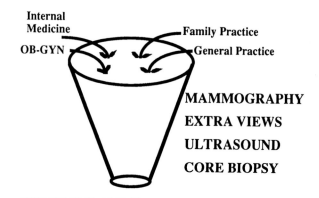

FIG. 7. Complete diagnostic workup of a breast lesion. A good mammographic workup followed by necessary adjunctive methods should proceed in a logical stepwise fashion with a refined product available at the end—a definitive diagnosis.

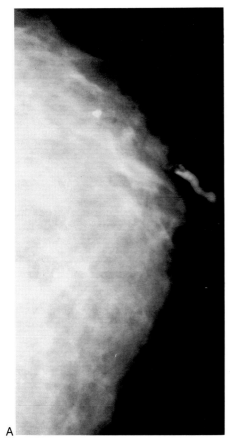
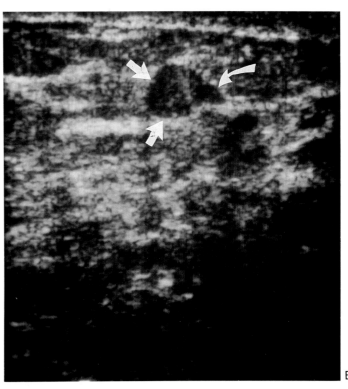

FIG. 8. Intraductal papilloma. **A:** Ductogram showing a nodular filling defect with a "tail" extending along the duct toward the nipple. **B:** Ultrasound image showing the same papilloma (*straight arrows*) and extension along the duct (*curved arrow*).

form the biopsy. This is sometimes impossible to overcome in spite of repeated reassurances. In such cases, the region is stereotactically biopsied rather than having the patient go on to surgical biopsy.

Providing the best prebiopsy diagnosis through the use of additional mammographic views and other adjunctive methods (e.g., ultrasound, ductography) is essential for successful core biopsy. Ruling out benign or artifactual lesions (e.g., superimposed fibroglandular tissue) eliminates chasing ephemeral targets or biopsying nonexistent lesions. More importantly, a firm or at least a short differential diagnosis before biopsy can be correlated with the subsequent histologic core diagnosis. Patients whose histologic diagnoses do not match the prebiopsy diagnoses become candidates for repeat biopsy. Not having a firm prebiopsy diagnosis to compare with the eventual core diagnosis increases the potential for false-negative core biopsy.

GUIDANCE SELECTION

Prebiopsy workup also helps the radiologist select the best imaging technique, either stereotactic mammography or ultrasound, for guiding the biopsy. Naturally, if the radiologist is not well versed in ultrasound

the inclusion of ultrasound in the workup of a mammographic lesion would not be as useful because this technique would not be considered for biopsy guidance. In this case, all biopsies would be performed using stereotactic guidance. However, even radiologists not highly skilled in ultrasound can use it to differentiate between solid and cystic lesions.

Ultrasound is, however, the preferred guidance technique for core biopsy at the BDCC because it is faster, is less uncomfortable for the patient, and utilizes no ionizing radiation. Therefore, it is an integral part of the workup of many breast lesions. (Guidance selection and ultrasound guidance are more completely covered in Chapter 13).

PREBIOPSY PREPARATION

Once the radiologist, technologist, and nurse become an experienced team, the radiologist does not need to be present until the patient has been positioned and prepped. By conferring with the radiologist, the technologist and nurse can usually handle all of the patient preparation while the radiologist attends to other patients and/or duties.

Generally, the BDCC nurse handles most of the

counseling, and the radiologist gets involved only at the patient's request (see Chapter 4). Some radiologists may prefer to counsel the patients themselves. Regardless of who counsels the patient, it is imperative to educate her as completely as possible. Patients at BDCC are informed that ultrasound biopsy may also be necessary to evaluate their lesions. Rebiopsy, usually percutaneous core biopsy but possibly surgical biopsy, could also be recommended. It should be emphasized to the patient that no biopsy method, including surgery, is perfect. The importance of follow-up, both clinical and radiologic, should also be stressed.

Although patient workup is directed by the radiologist, most of it can be handled by the technologist. A highly motivated, highly skilled technologist is invaluable for both patient workup and the biopsy itself (see Chapter 5). Even with such a technologist, however, it is still essential that the radiologist and the technologist confer before, during, and after the workup. Together they must ensure that all questions regarding location and number of lesions, lesion makeup, and expected biopsy approach are answered before the patient is set up for the actual biopsy.

THE EQUIPMENT

Both adapted add-on and dedicated stereotactic equipment are available. All biopsies at the BDCC are

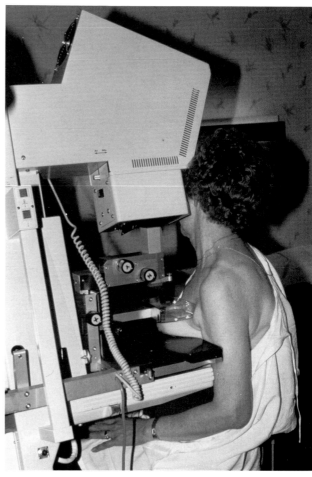

FIG. 10. An "add-on" stereotactic unit. The patient must actively pull her head away from the tube housing as it goes through its 30° arc, creating the potential for breast movement. In addition, it is difficult for the patient to hold the seated position for 30 to 40 minutes without slouching or making other physical adjustments secondary to fatigue. (From Parker and Jobe, Ref. 9a, with permission.)

performed with a dedicated unit (Fischer Mammotest; Fisher Imaging Corporation, Thornton, Colorado) (Fig. 9 in this chapter and Fig. 3 in Chapter 5) because dedicated recumbent systems largely eliminate the drawbacks of the add-on units (Fig. 10). A dedicated recumbent stereotactic system is also available from LORAD (LORAD Medical Systems; Danbury, Connecticut) (Fig. 11).

With recumbent tables the patient lies prone, with her breast placed through an opening at the head of the table (Fig. 12). The recumbent position virtually eliminates the problems with patient movement and vasovagal reactions which plague the add-on units. The stereotactic and biopsy apparatus, x-ray tube, and compression plate are all beneath the table, free of encumbrances and out of sight so that the patient is not subjected to watching a needle pierce her breast (Fig. 12). The actual biopsy site and the biopsy needle are

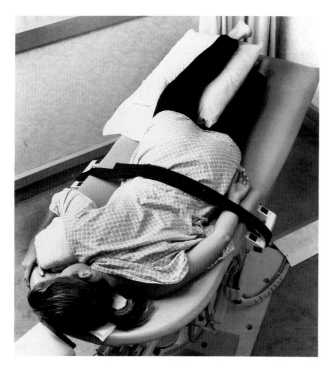

FIG. 9. Fischer Mammotest dedicated stereotactic unit. The patient lies prone on the table, and her breast protrudes through an opening in the table. (Courtesy of Geoffrey Wheeler.)

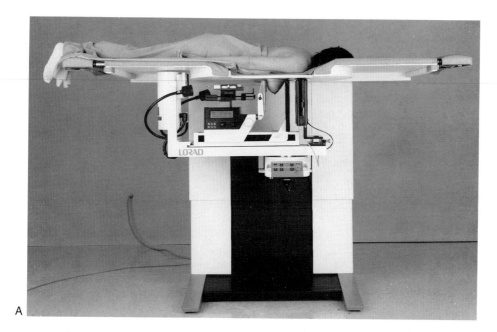

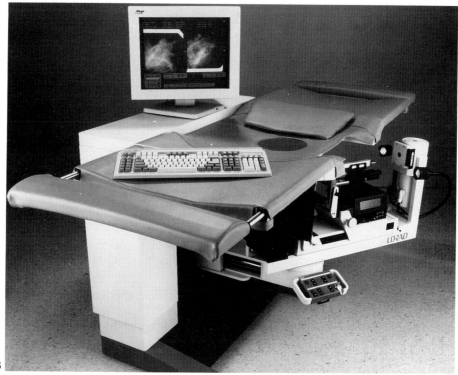

FIG. 11. LORAD dedicated prone stereotactic unit. **A:** The hole for breast placement is in the center of the table, which allows the patient's feet to be placed at either end. This makes a caudal-cranial approach possible. **B:** Working space in the craniocaudal approach is more limited than with the Mammotest, since access to the breast is available from only one side. (Courtesy of LORAD Medical Systems, Danbury, Connecticut.)

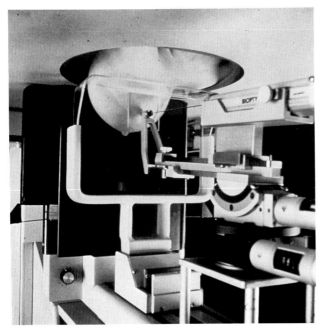

FIG. 12. A dedicated prone stereotactic approach allows an unrestricted working area out of sight of the patient. The biopsy gun can be solidly locked into the holder, eliminating the possibility of unwanted gun or needle angulation. (From Parker et al., Ref. 1, with permission.)

less likely to become contaminated with dedicated systems than with add-on units. The dedicated housing designed to hold the biopsy device firmly in place eliminates any unwanted needle movement or angulation. Although the dedicated systems can accommodate both aspiration needles and automated biopsy devices, all patients at the BDCC are biopsied using automated 14 gauge needles. (Fine-needle aspiration biopsy is covered in Chapter 9.)

THE TECHNIQUE OF STEREOTACTIC BIOPSY

The first step in the stereotactic biopsy procedure involves obtaining a scout image in the craniocaudal, mediolateral, or lateromedial projection (Fig. 13). (With the LORAD unit a caudocranial approach can also be used.) After the scout view has been developed and shows the lesion within the aperture in the compression plate, stereo views are obtained and placed on the adjacent digitizer (Fig. 14). A hand-held computer "mouse" is activated at the center of the lesion and at reference coordinates in each stereo view (Fig. 15). The digitizer prints out the horizontal and vertical coordinates along with a depth. The lesion's coordinates are then dialed into the main unit. The skin is anesthetized, a skin nick is made with a scalpel, and cores are obtained. Additional details pertaining to each of these steps are described below.

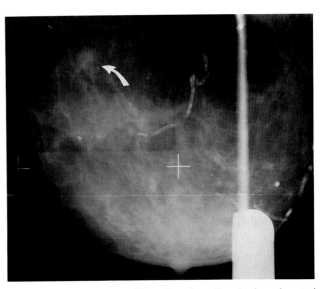

FIG. 13. Initial scout film showing the lesion (*arrow*) within the aperture in the compression plate.

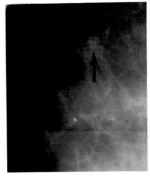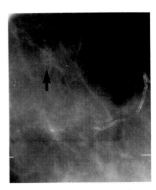

FIG. 14. Stereotactic scout views with intended biopsy points marked on the lesion in each view (*arrows*).

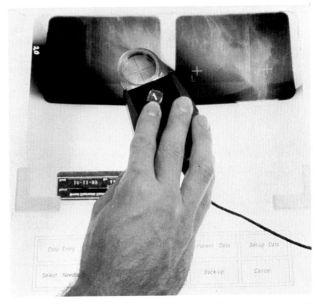

FIG. 15. Digitizer. The lesion is located in each view with the "mouse," and coordinates are generated. (From Parker and Jobe, Ref. 9a, with permission.)

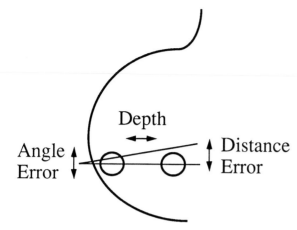

FIG. 16. Schematic representation of increasing distance error for given angle error as the depth of the lesion increases.

distance error increases for a given angle error the further the needle has to travel to the lesion (Fig. 16). Therefore, a short skin-to-lesion distance will provide more accurate targeting even if a small angle error exists. Also, approaching the lesion using the shortest distance leaves more breast tissue between the lesion and the back of the breast. This allows for easy excursion (2.3 cm) of the biopsy needle. Finally, since some breast surgeons excise the biopsy tract when performing breast conservation surgery, the shortest approach to the lesion is especially important in patients with malignant lesions who subsequently undergo lumpectomy.

The location of the needle tract can also alter the surgeon's approach to the lumpectomy. When possible, many surgeons prefer to use a periareolar approach, which blends the incision into the border between the areola and the breast, because it creates a better cosmetic result. A skin entry point (for core biopsy) approximately 1 cm from the areolar margin allows excision of the needle tract so that the skin margins are at the border of the areola. Other surgeons want the radiologist to use a skin entry point along the radial line equidistant from the areola. Every surgeon's approach to lumpectomy and needle tract excision is at least slightly different. It is therefore prudent for radiologists to familiarize themselves with the local surgical community's and referring surgeons' standards so that the appropriate skin entry point can be selected.

Details of the entire procedure from the nurse's, technologist's, and radiation physicist's points of view are discussed in Chapters 4, 5, and 6, respectively. Details of digital stereotactic technique and the use of an automatic alignment device are discussed in Chapter 14.

The view chosen for the scout film depends upon the lesion's location within the breast as determined by the prebiopsy workup. The projection (e.g., mediolateral) that provides the shortest distance to the lesion is preferable for several reasons. Using a short distance to the lesion improves targeting accuracy because the

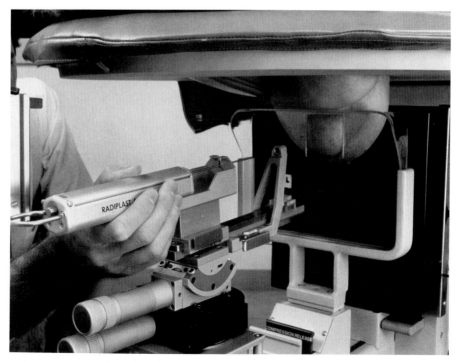

FIG. 17. Biopsy gun and housing. The gun must be advanced flush with the forward side of the housing and then fixed securely with the thumb screw.

Once it is clear that the patient is in the appropriate position for the shortest approach to a lesion, the biopsy gun is locked into place in its dedicated housing (Fig. 17). The coordinates are dialed into the main unit, aligning the gun and needle on the proper trajectory (Fig. 18). The needle and gun assembly is advanced to a point just short of the skin so that it is clear exactly where the skin anesthetic should be placed (Fig. 19). Mixing sodium bicarbonate with the local anesthetic to neutralize the solution ensures that it does not sting when injected. With stereotactic biopsy only a small amount of skin anesthesia is administered. Deep instillation of local anesthetic is generally not advisable. It can obscure soft tissue lesions, since both are of water density. Although deep anesthetic does not obscure clustered microcalcifications, it may move them, which then necessitates relocalization (Fig. 20). Using less anesthetic with stereotactic biopsy than with ultrasound biopsy is usually not a problem because breast compression itself provides a degree of anesthesia. (The instillation of deep anesthetic for ultrasound-guided biopsy is covered in Chapter 13.)

After anesthetizing the skin, the radiologist can then advance the needle into the skin wheal slightly, leaving an indentation. The indentation can be used for guiding the scalpel to the exact point where the needle will enter the skin. A skin nick just large enough to admit the 14 gauge needle is sufficient (Fig. 21). If a skin nick is not made and the needle is advanced through virgin skin, the skin hinders the action of the outer cannula and several passes are required before the skin entry

point is loosened up enough to obtain consistent cores. It is helpful, as well, to wiggle the tip of the scalpel back and forth just inside the skin when making the nick. This helps break up the subcutaneous tissues, again allowing easier passage of the needle and unrestricted, rapid action of the outer cannula. After the nick is made, the needle is advanced to the designated depth and repeat stereo views are obtained (Fig. 22). The needle is then withdrawn 5 mm to position the sample notch properly for the most accurate tissue acquisition (see Chapter 6, especially Fig. 16).

If the needle is in danger of striking the back breast support when the coordinates are digitized, a negative stroke margin warning is elicited. If the computer reads out a negative stroke margin, then 3 mm are added to it as a safety margin. For example, if the stroke margin is -4 mm, then the needle tip would be withdrawn 7 mm before the gun is fired.

After the needle is withdrawn the appropriate distance, the gun is fired (Fig. 23). Then a set of postfire stereo views is obtained to document the needle traversing the lesion (Fig. 24). At least five passes are made to obtain representative samples throughout the lesion. The other four points routinely targeted include the peripheral four quadrants (Fig. 25). Additional stereotactic documentation of the other four passes is not necessary if the initial pre- and postfire views of the center of the lesion show accurate targeting.

Naturally, if the targeting is not accurate, relocalization is required. The pre- or postfire stereo image is placed on the digitizer, and the new location of the

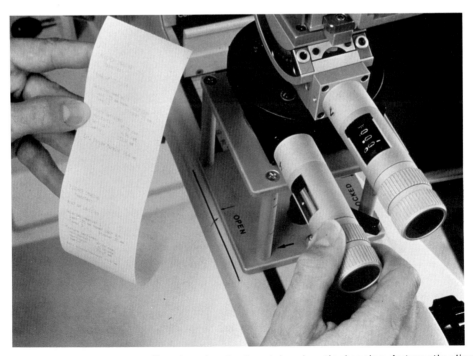

FIG. 18. Coordinates are manually entered on horizontal and vertical scales. Automatic alignment mechanisms will soon be available (see Chapter 14).

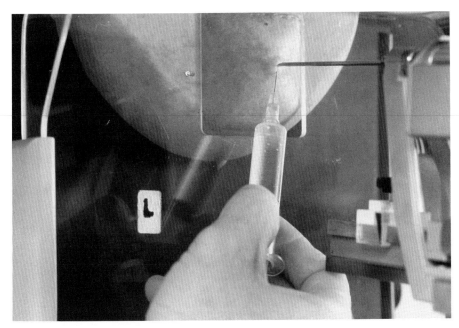

FIG. 19. A skin wheal is raised with anesthetic. The tip of the biopsy needle is used to guide the placement of the wheal. (From Parker et al., Ref. 11a, with permission.)

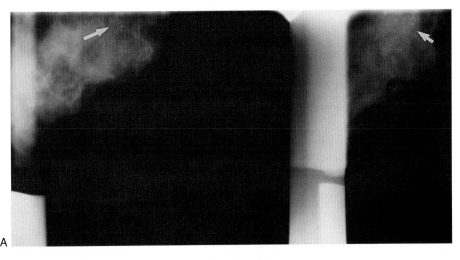

A

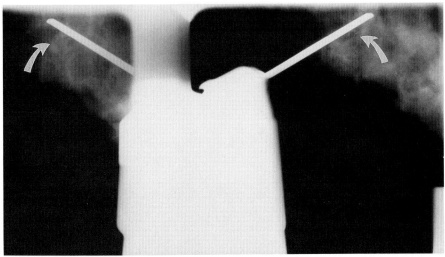

B

FIG. 20. Movement of clustered calcifications after the instillation of deep anesthetic. **A:** Stereotactic scout view demonstrating a small cluster of calcifications near the top of the compression plate aperture (*arrows*). **B:** Postfire views obtained after the instillation of local anesthetic show that calcifications have moved anteriorly (*arrows*).

71

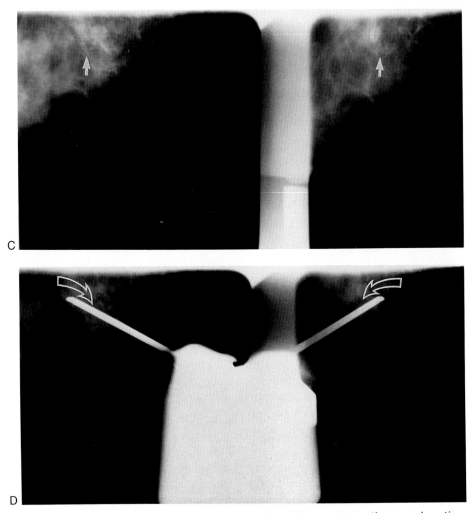

FIG. 20. (*Continued*) **C:** Repeat stereotactic scout view demonstrates the new location of the calcifications (*arrows*). **D:** Final postfire views show accurate targeting of the calcifications in their new location (**arrows**). (From Parker et al., Ref. 7, with permission.)

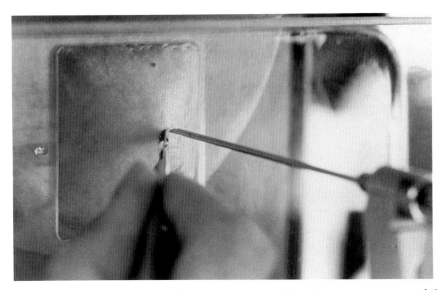

FIG. 21. A nick made in the skin wheal is just large enough to allow easy passage of the needle through the skin.

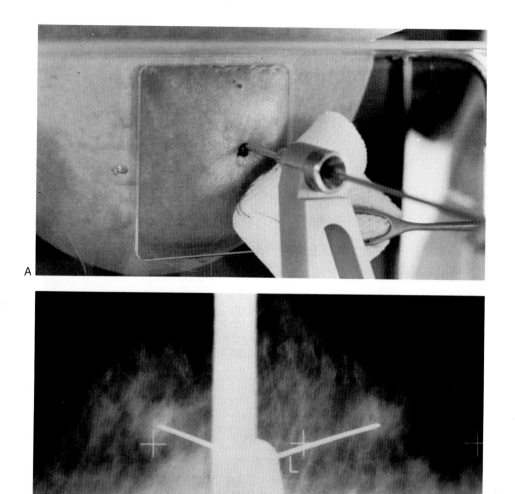

A

B

FIG. 22. A: The needle is advanced through the skin nick to the designated depth. On subsequent passes to peripheral parts of the lesion, the nick must be carefully moved to line up with the new needle trajectory. (From Parker et al., Ref. 11a, with permission.) **B:** Prefire stereotactic views showing the needle poised symmetrically over the lesion in both views indicate accurate targeting. (From Parker et al., Ref. 1, with permission.)

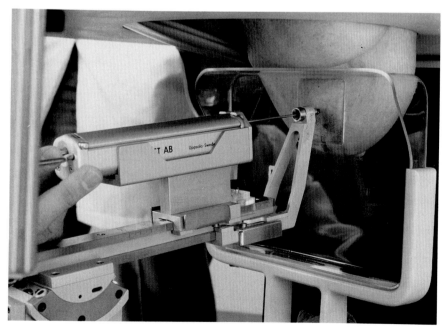

FIG. 23. After the prefire stereotactic views are obtained, the gun assembly and needle are withdrawn 5 mm and then fired. (From Parker and Jobe, Ref. 9a, with permission.)

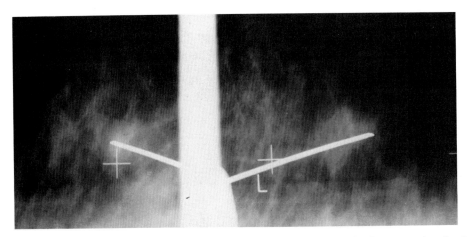

FIG. 24. Postfire stereotactic views demonstrating the needle symmetrically traversing the lesion in both views indicate successful targeting. (From Parker et al., Ref. 1, with permission.)

lesion is generated (Fig. 26). The biopsy apparatus does not need to be removed, and stereo scout views need not be repeated. It is imperative that relocalizations be carried out until pinpoint accuracy has been achieved and documented (Fig. 27). Potential pitfalls of stereotactic localization and the resulting biopsy errors are discussed in detail in Chapter 6.

Occasionally, a reference cross hair may be obscured on the pre- and postfire views. To locate the exact position of the obscured cross hair, one can draw a line horizontally through the remaining cross hairs. The line is marked at the known distance between the cross hairs to reproduce the obscured cross hair (Fig. 28).

Some radiologists believe that it is important to limit the number of passes to reduce morbidity (6,8,13). This concern is unfounded. As many as twenty 14 gauge passes have been completed in patients at the BDCC without creating infection, hematoma, or mammo-graphic pseudolesions. Ensuring adequate sampling of the lesion outweighs any theoretical concern for increased morbidity. This is especially true in cases of granular microcalcifications, as noted earlier, where the disease process may not be inherently related to those calcifications. In such cases, 10, 15, or even 20 cores through two or three separate skin nicks can safely be obtained throughout the region of interest to prevent a potential false-negative result.

All samples from the same lesion are placed in one sterile specimen cup with a *small* amount of physiologic saline (Fig. 29). Once samples from each lesion are collected, 10% formalin is added to fix the core tissue. Naturally, each pathologist who reads core specimens may want the radiologist to adjust specimen handling to meet the protocol of the pathology laboratory. Again, as with surgical standards, pathologic standards should be established jointly.

Specimen radiography of breast cores can document

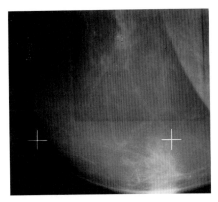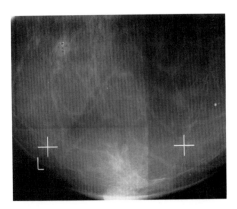

FIG. 25. Spray pattern of biopsy targets within a lesion. The distance that the four peripheral points are placed from the lesion center varies according to lesion size. Larger lesions require greater distances. If the peripheral points are much more than 5 mm from the lesion's center, it is not possible to move the skin nick to meet the needle. In such cases one or more additional nicks may be required.

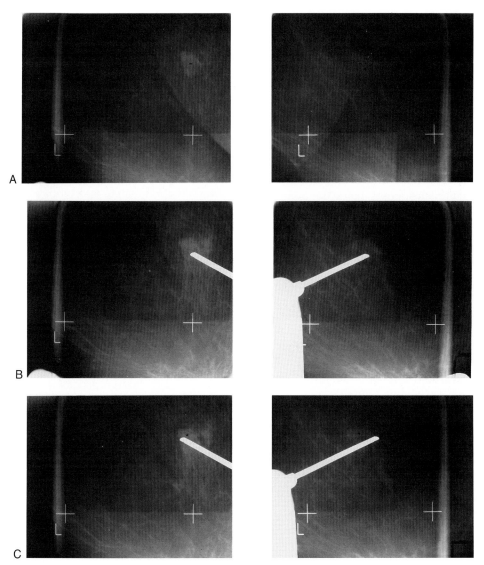

FIG. 26. Slightly inaccurate targeting requiring relocalization. **A:** Stereotactic scout view of the targeted lesion. **B:** Prefire stereotactic views. **C:** Postfire stereotactic views demonstrate that the needle has traveled slightly anteriorly, through the anterior portion of the lesion. A new center point has been marked for relocalization.

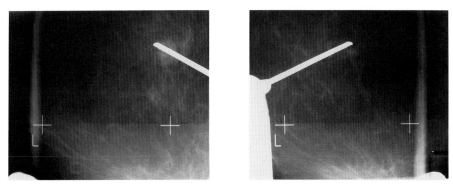

FIG. 27. Final postfire views, from the same case as in Fig. 26, demonstrate pinpoint accuracy in targeting the center of the lesion.

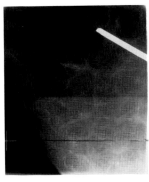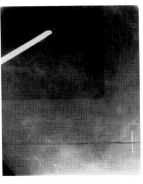

FIG. 28. Obscured reference cross hairs on postfire views used for relocalization. A straight line has been drawn through the two remaining outside cross hairs. The known distance between cross hairs is measured along this line to permit marking of the location of the obscured cross hairs. This allows the digitization to proceed as usual.

accurate targeting of lesions with microcalcifications (Fig. 30) (see Chapter 5). This is probably best done while the patient is still in position on the stereotactic table. In the rare case that calcifications are not seen on the specimen radiograph, additional samples can be taken immediately until specimen radiography reveals calcifications within the subsequent cores.

Occasionally, skin calcifications mistaken for paren-

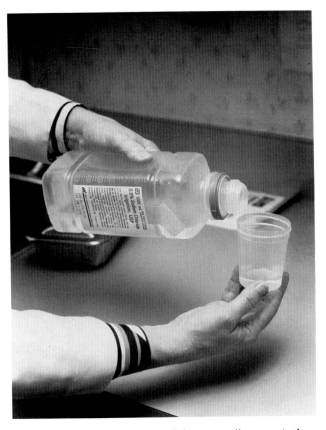

FIG. 29. Specimen cup containing a small amount of saline for the initial placement of core specimens.

chymal calcifications are scheduled for stereotactic biopsy. The resulting stereo coordinates would reveal that the calcifications are in the skin, and the biopsy could be canceled. A stroke margin of − 20 mm or more (for the long-excursion gun) would indicate that the calcifications are in the skin on the far side, adjacent to the breast support. A depth coordinate that would place the needle within a few millimeters of the skin on the near side, adjacent to the compression paddle, would indicate that the calcifications are in the skin closest to the x-ray tube.

Stereotactic imaging and biopsy are possible on lesions seen in only one standard mammographic projection, another advantage of the technique (Fig. 31). With the lesion seen in only one projection, however, the approach first chosen may not provide the shortest distance to the lesion. Once the stereo coordinates are obtained, it may become apparent from the depth coordinate where the lesion resides within the breast, and it can then be more confidently identified on the other view. If a different projection and skin entry point would place the lesion considerably closer to the skin than would the first approach, the patient can be repositioned and the stereo process begun again using another projection. For example, a lesion seen well only in the mediolateral projection which results in a negative stroke margin when localized on the digitizer actually resides in the lateral aspect of the breast. In this case the patient could be repositioned for a lateromedial approach so that the biopsy could proceed through a skin entry point much closer to the lesion.

After the biopsy, manual pressure is held over the biopsy site, including the needle tract and the lesion, for at least five minutes. Prolonged oozing of blood during the biopsy naturally requires longer compression. A compression bandage is then applied to the breast. (Postbiopsy care and counseling are covered in Chapter 4.)

The patient returns on the following day to be reexamined by the nurse. If the patient or nurse has any questions or concerns, the radiologist can speak to the patient at this time. If there is then any clinical concern, an ultrasound examination can rule out the existence of a hematoma. It is inappropriate to assume that there is a hematoma on the basis of physical examination alone. Ultrasound has demonstrated that virtually all cases of postbiopsy lump at the BDCC were due to edematous breast tissue without a discrete mass or fluid collection. Ecchymosis and some interstitial bleeding are not uncommon. No significant infection or other complication has been reported using this or similar procedures (2,7,8,14).

If no problems are encountered on the follow-up clinical visit, the patient is advised to resume normal activities. Patients at the BDCC return in six months for a follow-up unilateral mammogram to ensure that there

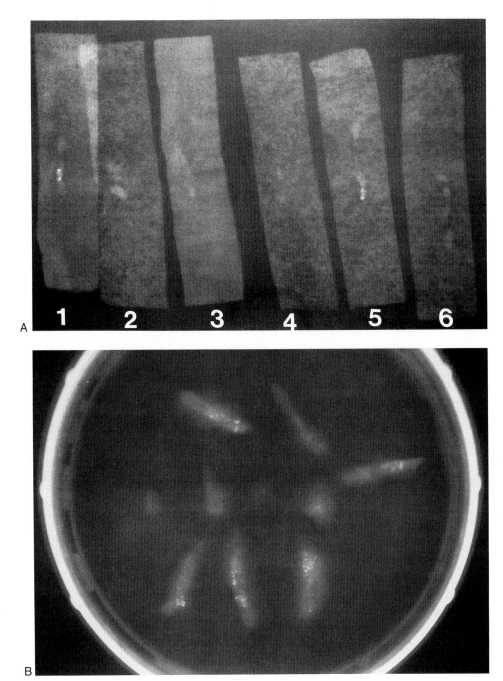

FIG. 30. Specimen radiography of cores. **A:** Individual cores have been placed on individual strips of sterile tissue paper and x-rayed. The first and fifth cores contain calcifications. **B:** The preferred method of specimen radiography at the BDCC involves pouring the small amount of saline and cores into the lid of the specimen cup. The excess saline is aspirated from around the cores, and then the lid is x-rayed. After the specimen radiograph is obtained, the cores are rinsed back into the specimen cup with formalin. This method ensures minimal handling and reduces physical trauma to the cores.

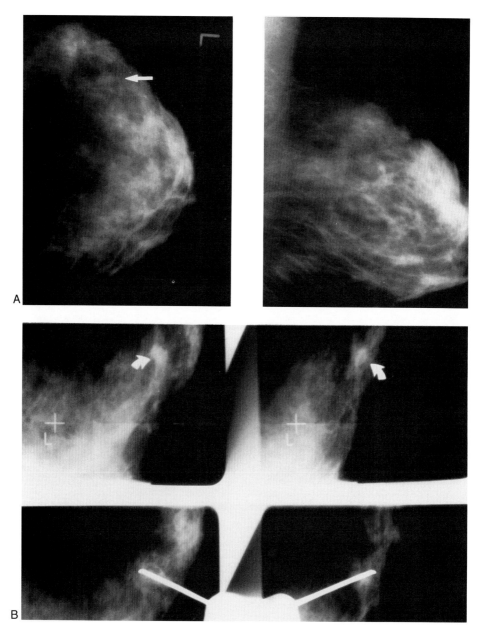

FIG. 31. Stereotactic biopsy of a lesion seen in only one projection. **A:** Ill-defined density seen only on the craniocaudal view (*arrow*). **B:** Stereotactic scout view (*top*) reveals that the density (*arrows*) persists in both views and therefore is not superimposed normal fibroglandular tissue. The postfire stereotactic view (*bottom*) demonstrates accurate targeting of the lesion. The histologic diagnosis was infiltrating ductal carcinoma. (From Parker et al., Ref. 7, with permission.)

has been no change. Some radiologists use a 4-month follow-up regimen, and some will undoubtedly recommend a 12-month follow-up. Regardless of the interval, if the findings remain stable at follow-up and continue to fit the needle-core diagnosis, the patient can then return to routine screening.

THE TEAM APPROACH

As the stereotactic biopsy team becomes experienced and comfortable with the procedure, the time required for the biopsy decreases. With an experienced team, the average total procedure time is approximately 30 to 40 minutes. The radiologist's time makes up approximately 15 minutes of the total procedure time. In light of this, patients are scheduled one hour apart at the BDCC. This allows enough time to finalize the prebiopsy workup; counsel, position, and prep the patient; perform the biopsy and postbiopsy care; review postbiopsy instructions; clean the biopsy room and apparatus; set up a new biopsy tray; and prepare the room for the next patient. Once the biopsy team is functioning smoothly, the radiologist need not get physically involved in a biopsy until the patient has been positioned and stereo scout images have been developed and placed on the digitizer. After successful targeting has been achieved and adequate tissue obtained, the radiologist can leave the patient in the capable hands of the remaining members of the biopsy team and return to other duties.

CONCLUSION

Stereotactic mammography allows pinpoint needle placement. With automated, long-excursion, large-gauge needles, this technique renders definitive histologic diagnoses with an accuracy equivalent to that of surgical diagnosis (7). Patient selection is similar to that for surgical biopsy. Additionally, cases of lower suspicion can be included when the patient's anxiety or the physician's suspicion is significant. Proper breast imaging workup must be performed before biopsy. Dogged pursuit of the lesion and postfire stereo views documenting the needle traversing the lesion are of paramount importance. Areas of widespread calcifications must be sampled extensively. It is also imperative that tissue samples be of superior quality and quantity. Only when both accurate needle placement and adequate tissue harvest have been assured can the radiologist consider the biopsy successful. If all of these requirements are met, stereotactic breast biopsy can be an expedient, cost-effective, and dependable alternative to surgical biopsy.

REFERENCES

1. Parker SH, Lovin JD, Jobe WE, et al. Stereotactic breast biopsy with a biopsy gun. *Radiology* 1990;176:741–747.
2. Dronkers DJ. Stereotaxic core biopsy of breast lesions. *Radiology* 1992;183:631–634.
3. Fajardo LL, Davis JR, Wiens JL, Trego DC. Mammographically-guided stereotactic fine-needle aspiration cytology of non-palpable breast lesions: prospective comparison with surgical biopsy results. *AJR Am J Roentgenol* 1990;155:977–981.
4. Mitnick JS, Vazquez MF, Roses DF, Harris MN, Gianutsos R, Waisman J. Stereotaxic localization for fine-needle aspiration breast biopsy. *Arch Surg* 1991;126:1137–1140.
5. Hopper KD, Baird DE, Reddy VV, et al. Efficacy of automated biopsy guns versus conventional biopsy needles in the pygmy pig. *Radiology* 1990;176:671–676.
6. Dowlatshahi K, Yaremko ML, Kluskens LF, Jokich PM. Nonpalpable breast lesions: findings of stereotaxic needle-core biopsy and fine-needle aspiration cytology. *Radiology* 1991;181:745–750.
7. Parker SH, Lovin JD, Jobe WE, Burke BJ, Hopper KD, Yakes WF. Nonpalpable breast lesions: stereotactic automated large-core biopsies. *Radiology* 1991;180:403–407.
8. Myer JE. Value of large-core biopsy of occult breast lesions. *AJR Am J Roentgenol* 1992;158:991–992.
9. Yankaskas BC, Knelson MH, Abernethy ML, Cuttino JT, Clark RL. Needle localization biopsy of occult lesions of the breast: experience in 199 cases. *Invest Radiol* 1988;23:729–733.
9a. Parker SH, Jobe WE. Large-core breast biopsy offers reliable diagnosis. *Diagn Imaging* 1990;12(10):91,94,95,97.
10. Tabar L. Early stage breast cancer: diagnosis and treatment. The state-of-the-art team approach. Presented at Lake Buena Vista, FL, September 17–19, 1992.
11. Holland R, Hendriks JHCL, Verbeek ALM, Mravunac M, Schuurmans Stekhoven JH. Extent, distribution, mammographic/histological correlations of breast ductal carcinoma *in situ*. *Lancet* 1990;335:519–522.
11a. Parker SH, Jobe WE, Yakes WF. Breast intervention. In: Castaneda-Zuniga WF, ed. *Interventional Radiology*. 2nd ed. Baltimore: Williams & Wilkins, 1992;2:1304,1305.
12. Stomper PC, Connolly JL. Ductal carcinoma *in situ* of the breast: correlation between mammographic calcification and tumor subtype. *AJR Am J Roentgenol* 1992;159:483–485.
13. Jackson VP, Reynolds HE. Stereotaxic needle-core biopsy and fine-needle aspiration cytologic evaluation of nonpalpable breast lesions. *Radiology* 1991;181:633–634.
14. Charboneau JW, Reading CC, Welch TJ. CT and sonographically guided needle biopsy: current techniques and new innovations. *AJR Am J Roentgenol* 1990;154:1–10.

Percutaneous Breast Biopsy, edited by
Steve H. Parker and William E. Jobe.
Raven Press, Ltd., New York © 1993.

CHAPTER 8

Stereotactic Breast Biopsy with "Add-on" Units

Laurie L. Fajardo

Mammography is currently the best method for detecting nonpalpable breast abnormalities. However, distinguishing between malignant and benign processes may be difficult based on mammography alone. Therefore, excisional biopsy with preoperative needle-wire localization is often recommended. The positive rate for surgical breast biopsies performed for mammographically identified nonpalpable abnormalities is, however, only 11% to 36% (1–11). There are significant costs related to diagnosing nonpalpable breast lesions, including patient morbidity and costs to health care insurers. In addition, a breast may show abnormal findings after a surgical procedure (most often, architectural distortion due to scarring) that can mimic a cancer and make interpretation of subsequent mammograms difficult. Mammographic needle biopsy, which addresses these shortcomings, is advocated as an alternative to surgical biopsy to diagnose some nonpalpable breast lesions.

"ADD-ON" VS. DEDICATED UNITS

Several manufacturers of mammography equipment are marketing stereotactic devices. Each of these devices has its own strengths and weaknesses. The costs range from $35,000 for systems that attach to existing mammography units ("add-on" stereotactic devices) (Fig. 1) to more than $150,000 for dedicated equipment specifically designed for stereotactic needle placement. Both add-on and dedicated stereotactic units can be used for either fine-needle aspiration biopsy or large-gauge core biopsy. When using add-on devices,

patients are seated while the procedure is performed. Advantages of the add-on stereotactic devices include lower costs, the ability to use the mammography unit for standard mammograms when the device is not attached, and the ability to biopsy deep breast lesions and axillary lymph nodes. These lesions may not be amenable to evaluation by stereotactic systems that require the patient to lie in the prone position during the procedure.

The major disadvantage of add-on stereotactic devices is the occurrence of vasovagal reactions. Although vasovagal reactions can occur with breast needle biopsies performed with the patient in the upright position, they are quite rare. Vasovagal symptoms occurred in approximately 1% of all patients biopsied at the University of Arizona Health Sciences Center (UAHSC) from 1988 to 1991, and all were alleviated with symptomatic treatment only. None required medication or the introduction of an intravenous line. As vasovagal reactions can often be triggered by psychologic distress, the following preventive measures can be helpful.

1. The temperature of the room in which the stereotactic breast needle procedure is performed should not be overly warm.
2. Closely attending to the patient and engaging her in conversation during the procedure directs her attention away from the procedure itself.
3. If the patient has confidence in the technologist and the radiologist performing the procedure, she will be more at ease. It may be helpful to schedule a short consultation visit with the patient a few days before the breast needle biopsy to explain the procedure and answer her questions.

L.L. Fajardo: Department of Radiology, Arizona Health Sciences Center, Tucson, Arizona 85724.

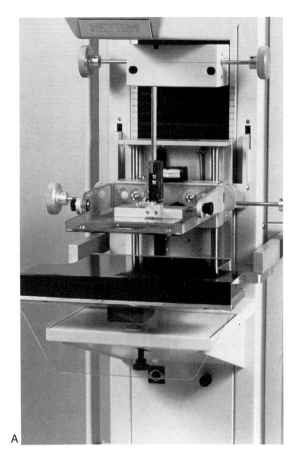

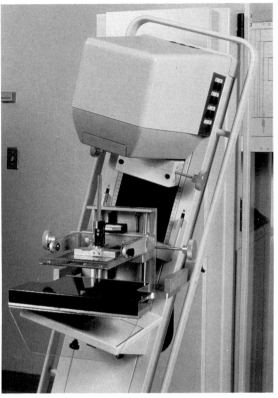

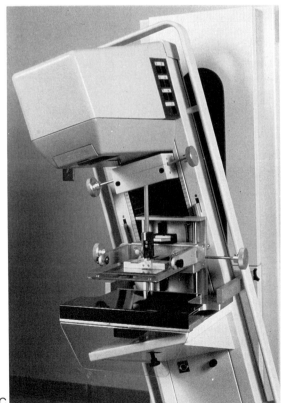

FIG. 1. A: Conventional screen-film mammographic system with the prototype ''add-on'' stereotactic device developed at the University of Arizona in place. **B,C:** A lock on the stereotactic device allows the C-arm of the mammography system to rotate +15° (**B**) and −15° (**C**) while the image receptor and the patient's breast remain stationary.

STEREOTACTIC LOCALIZATION

Stereotactic devices take advantage of the principle of triangulation. Calculation of the amount of deviation of the lesion on two views, obtained 30° apart, allows precise determination of the lesion's location in three dimensions (Fig. 2). Three-dimensional, Cartesian coordinates can easily be calculated using simple geometry from an image obtained with no angulation of the x-ray tube and two additional images obtained at +15° and −15° from the initial image (Fig. 3). The most recent generation of add-on stereotactic mammography devices utilizes a computerized light box and mouse-driven device to enter the stereotactic image information and automatically calculate the precise x, y, and z coordinates of a lesion within the breast. The newer generation of devices uses only the +15° and −15° oblique images to localize a breast mass.

After the three-dimensional location of a breast abnormality is calculated, the skin is prepared and a small amount (0.5 to 1.0 mL) of 2% lidocaine is injected. A 22 gauge fine-needle is placed, and stereotactic images

are repeated to confirm accurate needle placement. After this, gentle aspiration is initially performed. If fluid is aspirated, air and contrast agent are injected through the same aspiration needle and pneumocystography is performed. In general, the amount of contrast agent injected is slightly less than the amount of fluid aspirated.

If no fluid is aspirated, the lesion is assumed to be solid, and three to four fine-needle aspiration biopsies are performed. These samples are immediately stained and evaluated on site by the cytopathologists. If an adequate amount of cellular material was not obtained, repeat aspiration biopsies are performed. If the cytology specimens are negative and concur with the mammographic findings, no further intervention is performed and the patient is followed mammographically at 6, 12, and 24 months postbiopsy.

If the cytologic evaluation is suspicious or consistent with malignancy or if cytology is negative but the mammogram is suspicious, then four or five core biopsies are performed using a 14 gauge needle (Manan Medical Products, Northbrook, Illinois) and a long-throw (23

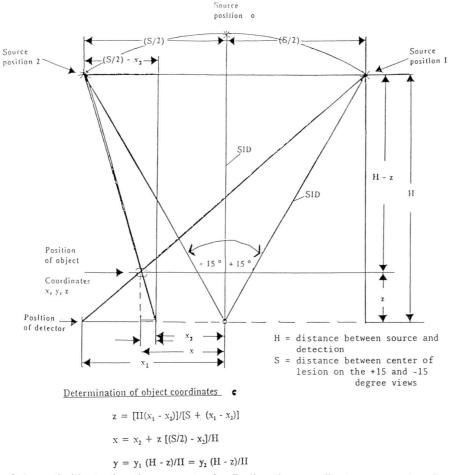

Determination of object coordinates

$$z = [H(x_1 - x_2)]/[S + (x_1 - x_2)]$$

$$x = x_2 + z [(S/2) - x_2]/H$$

$$y = y_1 (H - z)/H = y_2 (H - z)/H$$

FIG. 2. Schematic illustrating the geometry for finding the coordinates x, y, and z of an object (or breast lesion) from the coordinates x_1,y_1 and x_2,y_2.

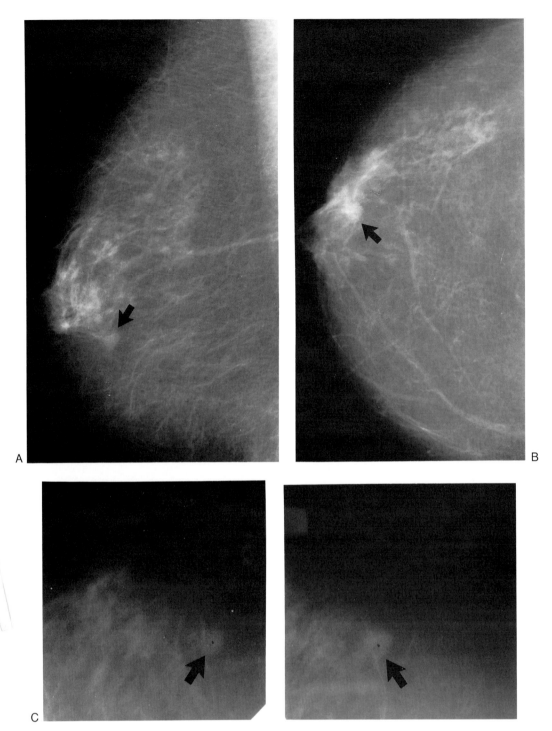

FIG. 3. A,B: Right oblique mediolateral (**A**) and craniocaudal (**B**) views of a 6-mm spiculate mass (*arrow*) in the 9 o'clock position of the periareolar area. **C:** Stereotactic images obtained at +15° (*right*) and −15° (*left*) of obliquity used for calculating the three-dimensional location of the mass (*arrow*). **D:** Repeat stereotactic images to document placement of the biopsy needle within the mass (*arrow*).

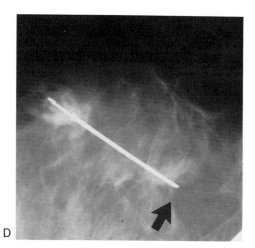

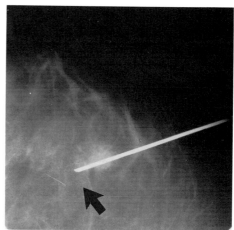

FIG. 3. *Continued.*

mm) Biopty gun (distributed by Bard Urological, Covington, Georgia; manufactured by Radiplast, Uppsala, Sweden).

Stereotactic core biopsy and stereotactic fine-needle aspiration biopsy techniques are discussed in detail in Chapters 7 and 9, respectively.

When initially instituting needle biopsy in the evaluation of nonpalpable breast lesions with add-on stereotactic units, a trial period of correlation between needle biopsy and surgical biopsy of 50 to 100 patients is recommended. This is especially important in practices where the pathologist is not familiar with breast disease and the radiologist is inexperienced in performing breast needle biopsy using an add-on unit. In such cases, a significant learning curve can be expected. In addition, the radiologist can use mammographic criteria to select cases that are likely to yield the best results.

THE STAGING OF BREAST CARCINOMAS

Early, limited experience at the UAHSC using add-on units to guide the biopsy of low-lying axillary lymph nodes has yielded encouraging results. Axillary lymph node biopsy can be used to stage breast masses or to evaluate for possible recurrence (Figs. 4 and 5).

When enlarged, dense axillary lymph nodes are seen mammographically in a patient with a suspicious breast mass, it is possible to evaluate both the mass and the lymph node(s) using stereotactic guidance. Figure 4

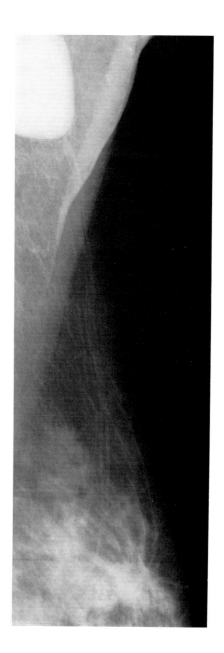

FIG. 4. Coned mammographic view from an oblique mediolateral projection showing a 1.5-cm spiculate mass in the upper outer quadrant of the left breast with an enlarged dense axillary lymph node. Stereotactic image-guided needle biopsy of both areas confirmed infiltrating ductal carcinoma with metastasis to the lymph node.

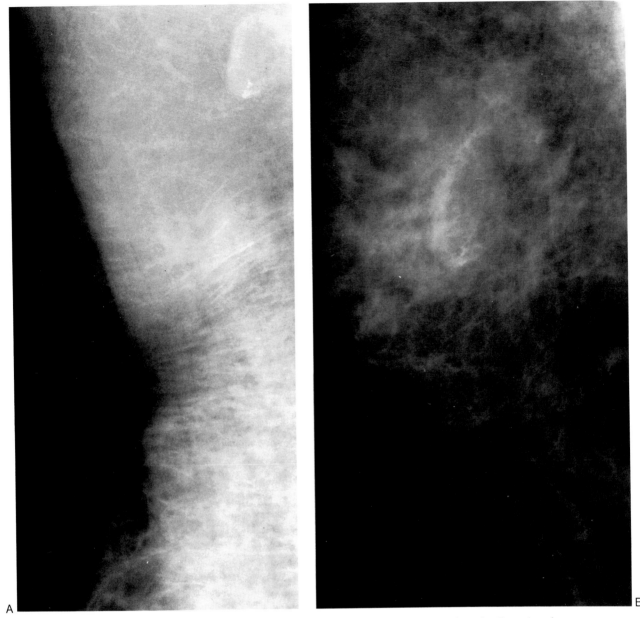

A

B

FIG. 5. A: Coned mammographic view from a right oblique mediolateral projection showing an axillary lymph node containing "microcalcifications." This patient had a prior history of right breast carcinoma (Stage I) that had been treated by lumpectomy and radiation therapy 22 months earlier. Although the mammogram showed no evidence of recurrence in the breast, there was concern that the lymph node might contain metastatic disease. Therefore, stereotactic mammographic image-guided biopsy of the node was performed. Calcifications were present in the core biopsy specimen, and the pathologic findings were consistent with dystrophic changes due to radiation therapy. There was no evidence of metastatic disease. **B:** The magnification image of the lymph node obtained after the biopsy shows a decrease in the number of calcifications in the node.

demonstrates the oblique medial lateral view of a patient with a spiculated mass in the upper outer quadrant of the left breast. Also note the enlarged, abnormal-appearing axillary lymph node. Under stereotactic guidance, fine-needle and core biopsy of both areas demonstrated that the mass in the breast was a cancer

and that there was extension of the cancer into the axillary lymph node.

Another patient (Fig. 5) who had undergone prior lumpectomy and radiation therapy for breast carcinoma was noted to have "microcalcifications" in an axillary lymph node. Although a breast lesion was not seen mammographically, there was concern as to whether the abnormal-appearing axillary lymph node represented recurrent carcinoma with nodal metastasis. Stereotactic fine-needle and core biopsy were performed on the lymph node using an add-on unit. Images obtained after the procedure demonstrated that the number of calcifications in the lymph node had diminished. Cytologic and histologic evaluation of the samples demonstrated that the calcifications were dystrophic and probably due to prior radiation therapy.

Positioning the patient for the sampling of axillary lymph nodes requires a skilled technologist and a cooperative patient. For these procedures, the add-on stereotactic devices are preferable, as it is unlikely that these areas could be adequately positioned for biopsy using a prone stereotaxic system. Women with kyphosis or severe arthritis may not tolerate the positioning required with either upright or prone stereotactic devices. Additionally, lesions located high in the axilla or deep within the breast may also be unsuitable for biopsy with stereotactic imaging. Biopsy in these cases might be accomplished with sonographic guidance (12) (see Chapter 13). In a minority of cases, surgical biopsy may be the only option.

SUMMARY

Add-on stereotactic devices provide an accurate, inexpensive means for evaluating nonpalpable breast lesions. In fact, deep upper outer quadrant breast masses are more easily accessed with an add-on than with a dedicated device because of the flexibility in positioning the patient with add-on systems. The minor disadvantage of add-on units, vasovagal reactions, is rare and self-limited and requires symptomatic treatment only.

Editors' Note: This chapter is included to present alternative techniques and viewpoints. Although we support attempts such as those described in this chapter to create nonsurgical alternatives to biopsy of breast lesions, we disagree with some of the equipment choices, techniques, and protocols described herein.

Regarding the disadvantages of add-on stereotactic equipment, we believe that patient motion and subsequent breast movement occur much more often with add-on units than with dedicated, prone units. We believe that patient movement is a result of the patient's inability to maintain her stationary position voluntarily while sitting or standing for an add-on stereotactic procedure. In addition, it is difficult to work with the automated core biopsy equipment in the tight quarters provided by add-on equipment.

Regarding fine-needle aspiration of cystic lesions, since we aggressively evaluate all lesions with ultrasound prior to any intervention, we do not aspirate simple cysts. If a cyst is noted ultrasonographically to

be complex, we attempt aspiration. We believe that pneumocystography is unnecessary in the age of high-quality, near-field ultrasound.

With respect to selecting a 14 gauge needle, it is important to realize that many manufacturers produce needles that fit into the Biopty gun. Although these needles superficially appear similar, it is crucial to evaluate the characteristics of each needle rather than using only one manufacturer's product. The reader is encouraged to review Chapter 2 for a more thorough discussion of needles.

Regarding the institution of breast needle biopsy in a given practice, we do not believe that a trial period of correlation between needle biopsy and surgical biopsy is necessary because data have already been published to document the accuracy of the technique. If a radiologist is comfortable with percutaneous needle biopsy techniques and with breast disease, there should be no reason to confirm initial percutaneous biopsy results with surgical biopsy. Naturally, the needle biopsy results must be closely evaluated and must agree with the prebiopsy mammographic diagnosis.

From our limited experience with the percutaneous biopsy of axillary lymph nodes, we believe that this procedure is accomplished much more easily using ultrasound guidance than using stereotactic guidance. The equipment, techniques, and protocols described in Chapter 7 (breast biopsy with dedicated stereotactic equipment and 14 gauge needles) and Chapter 13 (breast biopsy with ultrasound and 14 gauge needles) represent state-of-the-art percutaneous breast biopsy.

REFERENCES

1. Meyer JE, Kopanqs DB, Stomper PC, Lindfors KK. Occult breast abnormalities: percutaneous preoperative needle localization. *Radiology* 1984;150:335–337.
2. Gisvold JJ, Martin JK. Prebiopsy localization of nonpalpable breast lesions. *AJR Am J Roentgenol* 1984;143:477–481.
3. Proudfoot RW, Mattingly SS, Stelling CB, Fine JG. Nonpalpable breast lesions: wire localization and excisional biopsy. *Ann Surg* 1986;52:117–122.
4. Schwartz GF, Patchefsky AS, Feig SA, Schwartz AB. Clinically occult breast cancer: multicentricity and implications for treatment. *Ann Surg* 1980;191:8–12.
5. Hermann G, Janus C, Schwartz IS, Krivisky B, Bier S, Rabinowitz JG. Nonpalpable breast lesions: accuracy of prebiopsy mammographic localization. *Radiology* 1987;165:323–326.
6. Bigelow R, Smith R, Goodman PA, Wilson GS. Needle localization of nonpalpable breast masses. *Arch Surg* 1985;120:565–569.
7. Hoehn JL, Hardacre JM, Swanson MK, Williams GH. Localization of occult breast lesions. *Cancer* 1982;49:1142–1144.
8. Homer MJ, Smith TJ, Marchant DJ. Outpatient needle localization and biopsy for nonpalpable breast lesions. *JAMA* 1984;252:2452–2454.
9. Baker LH. Breast cancer detection demonstration project: five-year summary report. *Cancer* 1982;32:194–225.
10. Wilhelm MC, de Paredes ES, Pope T, Wanebo HJ. The changing mammogram: a primary indication for needle localization biopsy. *Arch Surg* 1986;121:1311–1314.
11. Landercasper J, Gunderson SB, Gunderson AL, Cogbill TH, Travelli R, Strutt P. Needle localization and biopsy of nonpalpable lesions of the breast. *Surg Gynecol Obstet* 1987:164:452–456.
12. Fornage BD, Faroux MJ, Simatos A. Breast masses: US-guided fine-needle aspiration biopsy. *Radiology* 1987;162:409–414.

Percutaneous Breast Biopsy, edited by
Steve H. Parker and William E. Jobe.
Raven Press, Ltd., New York © 1993.

CHAPTER 9

Stereotactic Fine-needle Aspiration Breast Biopsy

Laurie L. Fajardo

Both stereotactic FNAB and stereotactic core biopsy can be used to evaluate nonpalpable breast lesions. Finer needles cause less pain and less bleeding than do larger needles, require no skin incision before insertion, and are approximately $\frac{1}{20}$th the cost of most large needles. Cytologic analysis can be used to diagnose many nonpalpable breast lesions and to determine whether further diagnostic techniques, including core biopsy, are necessary.

For the greatest success with needle biopsies, close cooperation between the mammographer, a cytopathologist experienced in breast disease (1), the breast surgeon, and the surgical pathologist is important (2). Strict diagnostic criteria for both mammographic and cytologic examinations facilitates consistent patient management and follow-up (Table 1). It may be desirable to have all patients seen by the breast surgeon before any needle biopsy. In the event that a needle biopsy result warrants further surgical intervention, the patient will have already established a relationship with her surgeon. Also, since biopsy can slightly alter the palpable characteristics of a lesion, prebiopsy clinical examination may help the surgeon with subsequent clinical evaluations.

Core biopsy is described in Chapter 7.

INDICATIONS AND CONTRAINDICATIONS

Breast needle biopsy is indicated for three types of nonpalpable lesions.

Well-defined Masses That Appear Benign When the Patient, Referring Physician, or Radiologist Prefers Needle Biopsy to Follow-up Mammography

This situation commonly occurs with women who have a strong family history of breast cancer or when the mass is relatively large (i.e., larger than 1 cm) and no prior mammogram is available for comparison. In these cases, needle biopsy may diagnose an unexpected carcinoma, but far more often it documents the benign nature of the mass, which can then safely be followed by mammography without the need for surgical biopsy.

When it is suspected that a nonpalpable mass may represent a complex cyst, fine-needle aspiration is an excellent method to confirm the cystic nature of the mass. If fluid is aspirated, air and contrast agent are injected through the same aspiration needle and pneumocystography is performed. In general, the amount of contrast agent injected is slightly less than the amount of fluid aspirated. As long as complete evacuation of a complex cyst is confirmed, 14 gauge core biopsy is not indicated.

Indeterminate Lesions Exhibiting Some Characteristics Raising Suspicions of Carcinoma

Breast needle biopsy determines the benign vs. malignant nature of such lesions and may provide information for staging and guiding surgical therapy.

Lesions with Highly Suspicious Mammographic Findings

Fine-needle biopsy may confirm the presence of malignant cells. Core biopsy can confirm the presence or

L.L. Fajardo: Department of Radiology, Arizona Health Sciences Center, Tucson, Arizona 85724.

TABLE 1. *Mammographic and FNA cytology diagnosis*

Diagnosis	Mammographic findings	FNA cytology
0	Not applicable	Inadequate, acellular specimen
1	Benign Circumscribed, low density mass, or Round, uniformly dense microcalcifications, few in number (<5)	Benign Normal epithelial pattern of aggregates and cytologic features
2	Probably benign Low-density mass with partial border loss, or Round, uniformly dense microcalcifications (<15)	Atypical, benign Atypical with regard to cell groupings
3	Suspicious for malignancy Low-density mass with architectural distortion, or Circumscribed, high-density mass, or Microcalcifications of irregular shape and density	Suspicious Malignancy—suspect cells, not interpretable as carcinoma with absolute certainty.
4	Malignant Circumscribed, high-density or stellate, spiculated mass with architectural distortion, or Microcalcifications of irregular shape and density with architectural distortion	Malignant Cells indicative of malignancy

absence of invasion. This information can be used to plan whether inpatient or outpatient surgical biopsy can be performed, depending upon whether the need for lymph node dissection is known *a priori*.

Contraindications

Patients taking anticoagulants should not be biopsied until the anticoagulation has been reversed. For patients with artificial heart valves, prophylaxis similar to that utilized for dental work is used.

THE TECHNIQUE

After the location of a breast abnormality is calculated in three dimensions, the skin is prepared and a small amount of 2% (0.5 to 1.0 mL) lidocaine is administered. (Stereotactic localization using dedicated and "add-on" systems is covered in Chapters 7 and 8, respectively). At the UAHSC, four to six passes for fine-needle aspiration cytology are obtained with a 22 gauge, 3½-inch (8.9-cm) spinal needle (Sherwood Medical, St. Louis, Missouri). Depending upon the size of the lesion, the mammographer may wish to adjust the needle entry position slightly between passes to sample all areas of the mass. By having the mammography technologist apply suction to a 20-mL syringe attached to the needle by plastic tubing (K50L; Baxter Health Care, Valencia, California), the mammographer has both hands free to manipulate the needle up and down through the lesion. This should be done 10 to 20 times per pass with slight rotation of the needle between excursions. To obtain an adequate sample, the mammographer should also angle the needle 5° to 10° between

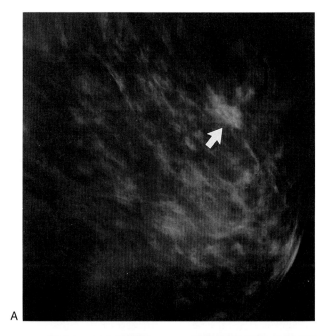
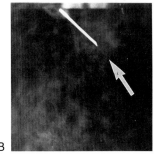
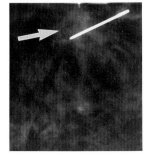

FIG. 1. A: Coned compression view (oblique mediolateral projection) of a 10-mm, irregular left breast mass (*arrow*). **B:** Stereotactic images confirming placement of the biopsy needle within the mass (*arrow*).

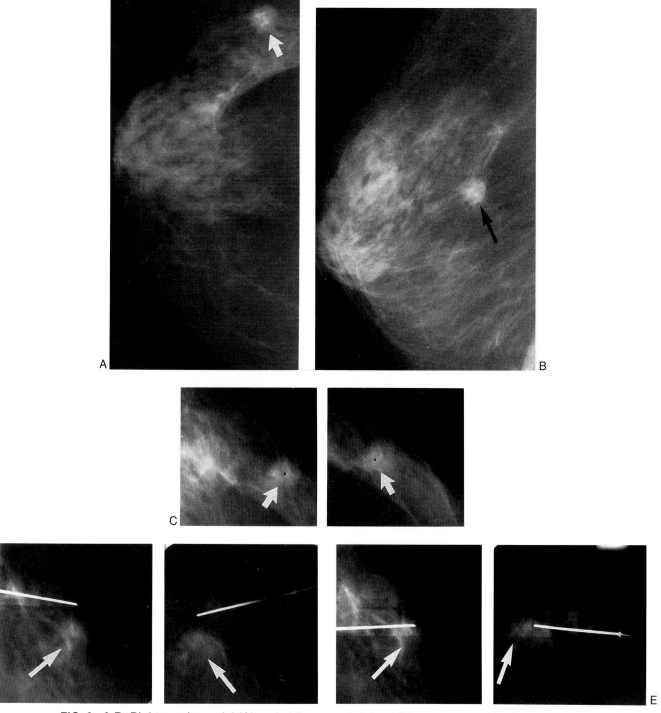

FIG. 2. A,B: Right craniocaudal (**A**) and oblique mediolateral (**B**) mammographic views showing a 1.2-cm mass (*arrow*) in the upper outer quadrant. **C:** Initial stereotactic images obtained to calculate the location of the mass (*arrows*). **D:** Repeat stereotactic images after the placement of a 22 gauge aspiration cytology needle show that the needle is located anterior to the mass (*arrows*) and requires repositioning. **E:** Stereotactic images obtained after repositioning of the needle confirm placement within the mass (*arrows*).

excursions in a fan-like fashion to avoid sampling the same needle tract repeatedly. In addition, the amplitude of the needle excursion should be greater than 1 cm (always greater than 5 to 6 mm) (3,4). Depending on the type of stereotactic device used for localization, this distance may need to be factored into the needle depth calculation. For example, if the center of a 10-mm lesion is calculated to be 22 mm from the skin surface, the needle guide should be adjusted so that the needle enters the breast to a depth of 27 to 28 mm to ensure passage through the entire lesion. Suction is released and the plastic tubing is disconnected from the needle before it is removed from the breast. After expressing the cytologic sample onto a frosted glass slide, the needle is flushed with 50% ethanol into a plastic tube for a cell block. The cytologic slides are immediately placed into 95% alcohol. The position of the biopsy needle should be confirmed and documented by at least one set of stereotactic images obtained during the aspiration procedure (Figs. 1 and 2).

Aspiration cytology biopsy specimens can be prepared and stained in the mammography suite by the cytotechnologist. They are preliminarily reviewed by the cytopathologist and immediately examined for adequacy and the presence of suspicious findings. If the cytology samples do not contain adequate ductal cells for evaluation, additional aspirates can be obtained.

If cells suspicious for malignancy are seen, 14 gauge needle cores can be obtained using a long-throw (23-mm excursion) Biopty gun (distributed by Bard Urological, Covington, Georgia; manufactured by Radiplast, Uppsala, Sweden). Core needle biopsy samples are placed in formalin. Histologic samples require 24 hours for fixation, processing, and interpretation. Core needle biopsy is not routinely performed on each patient at the UAHSC, however. Rather, the cytologic findings are used to determine whether a core biopsy is necessary.

Several types of needles have been used for breast aspiration and for core biopsy (5–13) (see Chapter 2). Ordinary spinal needles are an inexpensive choice for aspiration cytology. In about 4% to 5% of patients, adequate samples are not obtained in the initial passes and additional samples are needed. For repeat aspiration, it is useful to try a different type of needle. As a second choice, 22 gauge or 20 gauge 3½-inch (9-cm) "Westcott" style biopsy needles (MWN2003; Manan Medical Products, Northbrook, Illinois) can be used with good results. If widespread lesions are to be biopsied, additional passes are also necessary to ensure adequate sampling.

INTERPRETATION

A preliminary cytologic interpretation is made at the end of the procedure; the final diagnosis is available on the following day. Cytologic samples are evaluated for cellularity, cellular arrangements, nuclear-to-cytoplasmic ratio, and the characteristics of cell nuclei and nucleoli. Samples are classified on a scale of 1 to 4 as follows: 1 = benign; 2 = atypical, benign; 3 = suspicious for malignancy; 4 = malignant (Table 1) (10,14). Histologic core-biopsy samples are used to confirm a malignancy suspected from the cytologic specimen (cytologic diagnosis 3 or 4) and to determine whether a tumor is invasive.

THE ACCURACY OF FINE-NEEDLE ASPIRATION CYTOLOGY AND CORE BIOPSY

Several recent studies have compared the diagnosis of nonpalpable breast abnormalities using cytology with results from surgical biopsy (5,6,12). The sensitivity for fine-needle aspiration cytology has varied from 68% to 93%, and the specificity has varied from 88% to 100%. The frequency of acellular or inadequate breast cytologic specimens varies from 0% to 36% in these series. If immediate cytologic evaluation of aspirates can be performed, the occurrence of scanty or inadequate specimens can be largely eliminated.

Most interventional mammographers performing core breast biopsy use the automated Biopty device and 14 gauge needles (9). The sensitivity reported for core biopsy of nonpalpable breast lesions is 93%; the specificity is 98% (9). A few have used fine-needles (20 gauge) with automated biopsy devices and stereotactic localization. The sensitivity and specificity reported for this technique are 71% and 96%, respectively.

In most cases the accuracy of fine-needle biopsy correlates well with the findings on mammography. The most accurate cytologic yield is obtained from stellate masses with microcalcifications, well-defined masses, and stellate masses that were well depicted on mammography. Accuracy has been lower with ill-defined masses and clustered microcalcifications without an associated mass. The poorest results occurred with architectural distortions and radial scar types of lesions. These abnormalities frequently occupy relatively large areas in the breast and often are predominantly benign pathologically but can contain foci of carcinoma. If significant fibrosis is present, the cytologic samples may be relatively acellular, requiring a greater number of passes. Also, because of their size, radial scar lesions are difficult to sample in their entirety by either fine-needle aspiration cytology or core needle biopsy.

PATIENT FOLLOW-UP

At the completion of the biopsy procedure at the UAHSC, patients are given written instructions for postbiopsy breast care and follow-up. They are warned to expect slight bruising or discoloration at the biopsy site for 7 to 10 days. No serious bleeding complications have occurred. In a study of 100 patients biopsied with FNAB before breast needle localization and surgical biopsy (10), minor local hematoma was evident at the surgery in 35% of the patients. This did not, however, interfere with pathologic evaluation or receptor analysis.

Postbiopsy infection is rare to nonexistent. Should a local infection occur after needle biopsy, dicloxacillin, 250 to 500 mg orally every six hours (or q.i.d.), can be prescribed for patients not allergic to tetracycline. Alternately, nafcillin sodium (Unipen), 250 to 500 mg orally every four to six hours, can be prescribed for patients not allergic to penicillin. For very broad-spectrum coverage, ciprofloxacin (Cipro), 250 to 750 mg orally every 12 hours, can be used in patients who do not have a hypersensitivity to quinoline-type drugs. Treatment with ciprofloxacin is significantly more costly than is treatment with the other two agents.

PRACTICAL APPLICATIONS

Mammographic findings are combined with the results of fine-needle aspiration and core biopsies to manage patients with nonpalpable breast lesions at the UAHSC. When the core biopsy results indicate an invasive cancer, the patient undergoes a definitive inpatient surgical procedure with lymph node sampling. When an *in situ* carcinoma is suspected but not confirmed on core biopsy or when the cytologic findings are suspicious (cytologic diagnosis 3), the patient undergoes an outpatient breast biopsy. Rarely, these patients are found to have invasive carcinoma and require an inpatient surgical procedure.

If the findings of fine-needle aspiration biopsy are benign (cytology diagnosis 1 or 2) but the mammographic suspicion is high (mammographic diagnosis 3 or 4), the possibility of a sampling error must be considered. In such cases, a conservative approach is recommended (i.e., either repeating the needle biopsy or performing outpatient excisional biopsy). Further studies are needed to investigate the cost effectiveness of this approach.

Recommendations for follow-up with patients who have negative needle biopsy results is variable. The most common regimen involves follow-up mammography at 6, 12, and 24 months after the procedure. This protocol is identical to that used for mammographic follow-up of postlumpectomy patients. Any suspicious change on follow-up mammography of the previously biopsied nonpalpable breast lesion warrants reevaluation, either by repeat needle biopsy or by surgical biopsy. In one series of patients at the UAHSC whose management was based upon a combination of mammography and mammographic needle biopsy, 300 had benign biopsies and are in a follow-up regimen. Thirty-five percent of these patients have been followed for over two years. Of these, the overwhelming majority (greater than 85%) have shown no significant change on follow-up mammographic examinations. About 10% of these patients have demonstrated a decrease in the size of their breast mass on follow-up exams; in a smaller percentage (about 5%), the masses have disappeared. No missed cancers have yet arisen.

SUMMARY

Stereotactic fine-needle aspiration breast biopsy is best performed in a high-volume setting where the radiologist is experienced in performing the procedure and the pathologist is experienced in breast disease. Using core biopsy as an adjunct can be beneficial. Mammographic needle biopsy has the potential to reduce the number of surgical breast biopsies performed for mammographically detected lesions. This technique will become increasingly important in the management of breast lesions.

Editor's Note: This chapter is included to present alternative techniques and viewpoints. Although we support attempts such as those described in this chapter to create nonsurgical alternatives to biopsy of breast lesions, we disagree with some of the equipment choices, techniques, and protocols described herein.

We believe that the impression that finer needles cause less pain and less bleeding than do large needles is erroneous. With appropriate anesthetic, as described in Chapters 7 and 13, the discomfort experienced by the patient during core biopsy would be equal to or less than that experienced during FNAB without anesthetic. If an anesthetic is used for FNAB, then there is no difference at all in the potential discomfort. Some bleeding does occur with FNAB, as noted in the patient follow-up section of this chapter.

With regard to the fact that no skin incision is used for FNAB, the skin incision used for core biopsy heals virtually without a trace. Thus, there is no cosmetic difference between the two types of biopsy.

Regarding the cost of the needles used, automated core needles make up a minute portion of the overall biopsy charge. We do subscribe to the philosophy of cost containment. However, we believe that, overall, the increased cost of large needles is well justified by the histologic diagnoses provided by large needles. Also, regarding cost containment, we believe that initially using core biopsy eliminates the need for FNAB, which is frequently inconclusive and must be repeated or supplemented with core biopsy. The reader is encouraged to review Chapter 2 for a more thorough explanation of the advantages of core biopsy over FNAB.

The requirement for extremely close cooperation with pathologists and surgeons necessary with FNAB is largely eliminated with core biopsy. Requiring all patients to be seen by a breast surgeon before any needle biopsy is debatable. In many settings, this would significantly retard the implementation of needle biopsy of the breast, since the surgeons who initially see the patients would be more inclined toward open biopsy.

We believe that the equipment, techniques, and protocols described in Chapter 7 (breast biopsy with dedicated stereotactic equipment and 14 gauge needles) and Chapter 13 (breast biopsy with ultrasound and 14 gauge needles) represent state-of-the-art percutaneous breast biopsy.

REFERENCES

1. Cohen MB, Rodgers RPC, Hales MS, Gonzales JM, Ljung BME, et al. Influence of training and experience in fine-needle aspiration biopsy of breast: receiver operating characteristics curve analysis. *Arch Pathol Lab Med* 1987;111:518–520.
2. Hunter TB, Villar HV, Bjelland JC, Leong SPL, Barteau LL. Combined surgery-mammography conference: a way to optimize patient care. *AJR Am J Roentgenol* 1987;149:1081–1082.
3. Kreula J. A new method for investigating the sampling technique of fine needle aspiration biopsy. *Invest Radiol* 1990;25:245–249.
4. Kreula J. Effect of sampling technique on specimen size in fine needle aspiration biopsy. *Invest Radiol* 1990;25:1294–1299.
5. Fornage BD, Faroux MJ, Simatos A. Breast masses: US-guided fine-needle aspiration biopsy. *Radiology* 1987;162:409–414.
6. Evans WP, Cade SH. Needle localization and fine needle aspiration biopsy of nonpalpable breast lesions with use of standard and stereotactic equipment. *Radiology* 1989;173:53–56.
7. Hann L, Ducatman BS, Wang HE, Fein V, McIntire JM. Nonpalpable breast lesions: evaluation by means of fine-needle aspiration cytology. *Radiology* 1989;171:373–376.
8. Dowlatshahi K, Gent HJ, Schmidt R, Jokich PM, Biobbo M, Sprenger E. Nonpalpable breast tumors: diagnosis with stereotaxic localization and fine-needle aspiration. *Radiology* 1989;170:427–433.
9. Schmidt R, Morrow M, Bibbo M, Cox S. Benefits of stereotactic cytology. *Admin Radiol* 1990 Oct:35–42.
10. Fajardo LL, Davis JR, Wiens JL, Trego DC. Mammographically-guided stereotactic fine-needle aspiration cytology of nonpalpable breast lesions: prospective comparison with surgical biopsy results. *AJR Am J Roentgenol* 1990;155:977–981.
11. Parker SH, Lovin JD, Jobe WE, Luethke JM, Hopper KD, et al. Stereotactic breast biopsy with a biopsy gun. *Radiology* 1990;176:141–147.
12. Helvie MA, Baker D, Adler DD, Andersson I, Naylor B, et al. Radiographically guided fine-needle aspiration of nonpalpable breast lesions. *Radiology* 1990;174:657–661.
13. Jackson VP, Littman JS. Stereotactic breast biopsy precisely locates lesions. *Diagn Imaging* 1989 Nov:182–185.
14. McDivitt R, Stewart F, Berg J. Tumors of the breast. In: *Atlas of Tumor Pathology*. Washington, DC: Armed Forces Institute of Pathology; 1969:22–86.

Percutaneous Breast Biopsy, edited by
Steve H. Parker and William E. Jobe.
Raven Press, Ltd., New York © 1993.

CHAPTER 10

An Introduction to Breast Ultrasound

A. Thomas Stavros and Mark A. Dennis

THE GENERAL GOALS OF BREAST ULTRASOUND

Mammography is the proven and preferred screening method for breast cancer. Although not proven efficacious as a screening tool, breast ultrasound (BUS) is an effective diagnostic tool in the proper clinical setting (1–23).

The proper clinical setting in which to use BUS, however, is controversial. Japanese and German physicians broadly define appropriate indications and aggressively use BUS for diagnostic purposes (21,22,24). Most American radiologists more narrowly define indications for BUS and use it less aggressively as a diagnostic tool (2,4,6,8,17,23). In addition, American physicians rely more heavily on sonographers or radiographic technologists to perform breast sonography. This less aggressive use of ultrasound is most likely related to American radiologists' lower comfort level with "hands-on" ultrasound. Those who are facile and experienced in performing and interpreting real-time ultrasound tend to use diagnostic BUS aggressively. Relatively inexperienced radiologists are more likely to minimize its importance (24). Breast ultrasound is used in the United States primarily to determine whether known lesions are cystic or solid (2,4,6,8,17,23). Breast ultrasound can and should be asked to do more than that.

Breast ultrasound often can demonstrate cysts or solid nodules missed by mammography because of surrounding radiographically dense tissues (7,25–29). It can also show that a palpable abnormality or focal mammographic density is merely due to firm but normal fibroglandular tissues. Finally, ultrasound's real-time three-dimensional capabilities make it ideal for guiding needle localization, aspiration, and core biopsies (18–20,30–36).

Properly used, diagnostic BUS should be able to decrease the ratio of negative to positive biopsies by preventing unnecessary biopsy of cysts and palpable or mammographically asymmetric fibroglandular tissues with no decrease in sensitivity for cancer (and perhaps a slight improvement). Secondary benefits of this process include the detection of a few cancers missed by mammography and the elimination of unnecessary six-month follow-up mammograms. One of the costs of aggressive diagnostic BUS is that some fibroadenomas that never would have caused the patient problems will be discovered and possibly biopsied. In practice, many more biopsies are prevented by demonstrating cysts or fibrous tissue than are caused by finding fibroadenomas. Finally, the cost of these biopsies can be reduced if ultrasound-guided core needle biopsies replace open biopsies.

THE NORMAL SONOGRAPHIC BREAST ANATOMY

A tremendous amount of anatomic detail is visible sonographically. Sonographically identifiable normal structures include the skin, fat lobules, fibrous septae including Cooper's ligaments, other fibrous and fibroglandular elements, ducts, pectoralis muscle, ribs and costal cartilage, and pleura (16,21,25–27,37–39) (Figs. 1 through 5). Critics of BUS who claim that ultrasound does not have adequate resolution to evaluate the breast are mistaken. So many normal structures are identifiable sonographically, and their size and sonographic appearance are so variable, that it is difficult to be certain which of them are normal and which are

A.T. Stavros and M.A. Dennis: Radiology Imaging Associates, Breast Diagnostic and Counseling Centre, Englewood, Colorado 80111.

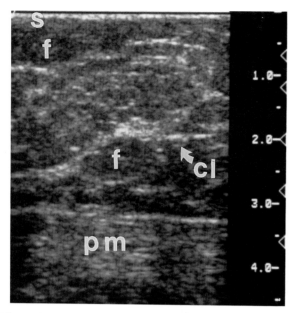

FIG. 1. Sonographic appearance of normal breast anatomy in a breast composed almost entirely of fatty tissue. The skin (s) and suspensory ligaments (cl) of the breast are highly echogenic. Time-gain curves are set to make the fat (f) appear a homogeneous medium-level echogenicity from the skin line to the pectoralis muscle (pm). The chances of mammography missing a lesion within such a fatty breast are very low. Ultrasound will be useful in characterizing mammographically visible lesions, but not in detecting palpable lesions which are undetectable mammographically.

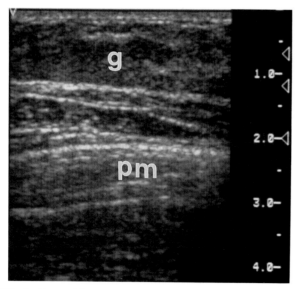

FIG. 2. Normal breast anatomy in a breast composed almost entirely of glandular tissue. Such an appearance can be seen in late adolescence and in the late second and third trimesters of pregnancy. Mammography showed uniform water density tissues throughout the breasts. Sonography shows a midlevel echogenicity throughout the mammary zones. This is similar to the echogenicity of the completely fatty breast in Fig. 1. It can be difficult to distinguish glandular from fatty tissue on sonograms without correlating mammograms. g, glandular tissue; pm, pectoralis muscle.

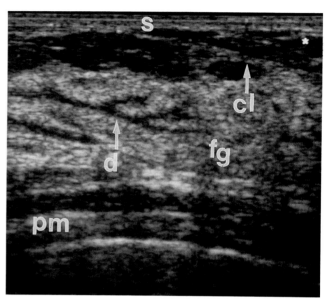

FIG. 3. Sonographic appearance of normal breast anatomy in a breast composed almost entirely of radiographically dense fibroglandular tissue. Only structureless homogeneously radiographically dense tissues were demonstrated on mammography. The skin (s) and suspensory ligaments (cl) are highly echogenic. The fibroglandular elements are also highly echogenic. Most of the echogenicity is due to fibrous elements, with ductolobular units being too small to resolve sonographically in most patients. Larger order ducts (d) 1 to 2 mm in diameter are demonstrable as linear branching structures of medium echogenicity within the surrounding, more echogenic fibrous elements. Ultrasound is able to show more structure within homogeneous water density tissue than can mammography. pm, pectoralis muscle; sqf, subcutaneous fat; fg, fibroglandular elements; d, mammary ducts.

not. The problem is demonstrating too many small structures of uncertain significance, not too few.

Besides nodules and normal tissues, sonography can demonstrate benign, enlarged, solid structures such as ducts and groups of ductolobular complexes. The appearance and size of these structures can vary markedly with time and between individuals. Ducts and ductolobular units may vary physiologically with heredity, age, menstrual cycle, exogenous hormonal therapy, pregnancy, and lactation, as well as with pathologic states. There is a continuous spectrum of size from normal structures to malignant lesions. For example, the prominence of visible lobular complexes increases in pathologic conditions such as adenosis. In florid adenosis, lobular complexes may be 3 or 4 mm in their largest dimension. Hundreds of such lobular structures may be visible throughout the breast (40–43). This creates a lower limit on the size of a sonographically visible solid structure that can be considered suspicious for malignancy. In the case of diffuse severe adenosis, solid structures less than 5 mm in maximum dimension are more likely to be benign hyperplastic lobular com-

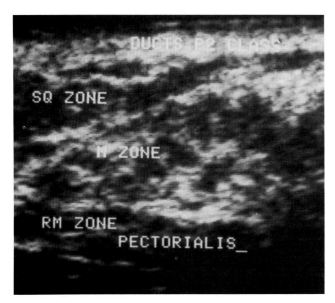

FIG. 4. Normal breast anatomy in a breast where involuted fatty lobules are interspersed with residual water density fibroglandular elements. The sonogram shows fat lobules that have midlevel echogenicity surrounded by highly echogenic fibroglandular elements. Both sonography and mammography can be difficult in such patients. It can be difficult to distinguish individual fat lobules from solid nodules on sonography, and there are enough residual dense breast tissues to obscure nodules on mammography.

plexes rather than cancers. Any of these small solid structures could hypothetically, however, represent a very small cancer. The shortcoming of sonography is not insufficient resolution to identify malignancy but is difficulty in distinguishing cancer from the myriad of normal and benign pathologic structures that ultrasound can demonstrate (Fig. 6).

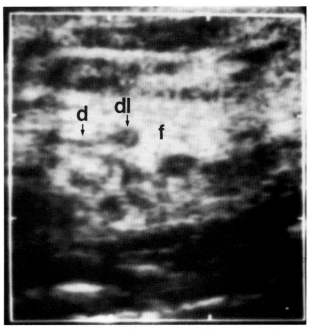

FIG. 6. Breast anatomy in a case of diffuse adenosis surrounded by dense fibrous tissue. Normal ductolobular units are generally too small to be resolved sonographically. In severe focal or generalized adenosis, however, coalesced ductolobular units may enlarge enough to be visible sonographically. These structures may be as large as 2 or 3 mm and may number in the dozens in focal adenosis or in the hundreds in generalized adenosis. Obviously, in such cases, we cannot consider solid structures less than 4 mm in diameter worrisome for malignancy. The sonogram shows an area of focal adenosis within an area of fibrous tissues. Branching ducts end in dilated structures probably representing conglomerations of enlarged ductolobular units. *f,* fibrous tissues; *d,* mammary ducts; *dl,* ductolobular elements (which may represent conglomerations of individual ductolobular units).

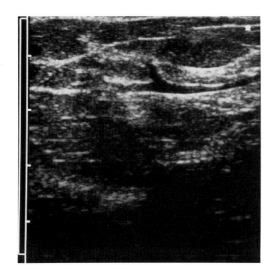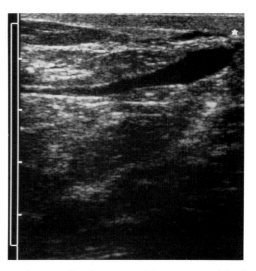

FIG. 5. Ductal ectasia. Fluid-filled ectatic ducts are frequently demonstrable sonographically. Such ectasia is most frequently seen in the lactiferous sinuses in the immediate periareolar area. Ductal ectasia may also involve lower order, more peripheral ducts. Ectatic ducts may be associated with secretions but more typically are asymptomatic. They are much more common in parous than in nulliparous women.

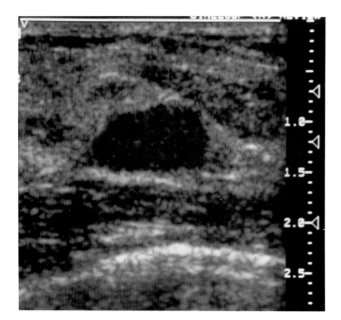

FIG. 7. Fibroadenoma surrounded by fibrous tissue. The mammogram showed dense lobulated tissues. The large palpable fibroadenoma could not be identified mammographically. The sonogram shows a highly conspicuous, well-circumscribed, homogeneous, well-transmitting, well-encapsulated mass surrounded by highly echogenic fibrous tissue. The marked echogenicity of the surrounding fibrous tissue dramatically improves the sonographic conspicuity of the lesion, while the similarity of the lesion's water density to that of the surrounding fibroglandular tissue obscures it mammographically.

Stromal fibrous tissues and fibroglandular elements are quite echogenic and appear white at sonography. Pathologic lesions such as simple and complex cysts, breast cancer, and fibroadenomas are generally hypoechoic and appear black to gray. When such hypoechoic lesions are enveloped within more echogenic fibrous elements, they are very obvious sonographically. Since fibroglandular elements and pathologic lesions are all water density, however, they may have similar or identical densities mammographically (8,26,29). Sonographically conspicuous pathologic lesions enveloped within fibrous tissues may, therefore, be mammographically invisible because of silhouetting by surrounding fibroglandular elements unless there are associated calcifications or architectural distortions. Because the mechanism by which sonography demonstrates lesions is so different from that of mammography, sonography can be quite complementary to mammography in "looking through" radiographically dense areas of the breasts (7,25–27,37) (Figs. 7 and 8).

THE INDICATIONS FOR BREAST ULTRASOUND

In the vast majority of patients, we use BUS only as an adjunct to mammography, performing a targeted examination on a localized area of a breast where there is either a focal clinical or mammographic abnormality (1–16,23,38). We perform more extensive whole-breast ultrasound or use ultrasound alone only under exceptional conditions.

The Specific Indications for Targeted Breast Ultrasound

1. Breast ultrasound should be used to evaluate palpable abnormalities when the mammographic findings in the area of concern are negative or nonspecific and when that area contains water density tissues (1–6,38). Lesions missed by mammography are usually surrounded by radiographically dense tissues (8,28,29). Breast ultrasound can look through those dense tissues to detect hidden cysts and solid nodules (7,25–27,37).

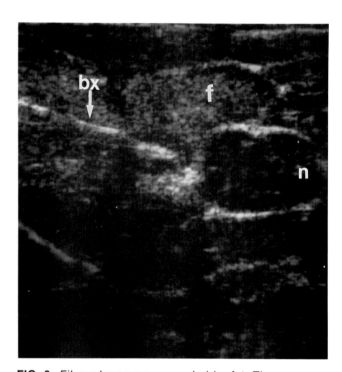

FIG. 8. Fibroadenoma surrounded by fat. The mammogram showed a highly conspicuous, well-circumscribed nodule. Sonography shows a very subtle, well-circumscribed, well-transmitting, homogeneous nodule slightly more hypoechoic than the surrounding fat lobules. The spatial resolution of sonography is good, but the contrast in echogenicity between the nodule and the surrounding fat lobules is low. Because of this lower contrast resolution, fat-surrounded nodules frequently have lower sonographic than mammographic conspicuity. In practice, this is not a major problem, since the mammogram that virtually always precedes sonography will detect all of these lesions. A discrete mammographic nodule 5 mm or more in diameter that cannot be demonstrated sonographically is almost always solid. Cysts of that size are too conspicuous to be missed on ultrasound. *n,* nodule; *f,* fat lobules; *bx,* core biopsy needle.

On the other hand, mammography is unlikely to miss palpable cancers in an area of the breast that is composed entirely of fat. Breast ultrasound of fat-surrounded lesions is not as accurate as BUS of lesions surrounded by echogenic fibroglandular elements (7,27,38,44–46). Breast ultrasound of a lump will, therefore, be useful in characterizing mammographically visible lesions, but not in detecting palpable lesions which are mammographically invisible (Fig. 9).

2. Breast ultrasound should be used to evaluate nonspecific mammographic lesions such as discrete nodules, less well-defined focal asymmetries, developing

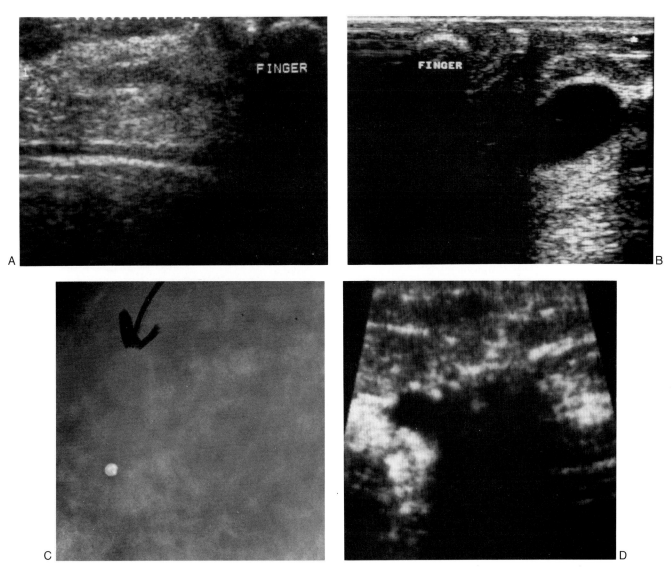

FIG. 9. When the indication for BUS is a palpable abnormality, it is important to palpate the abnormality while scanning to document its cause conclusively. **A:** Palpating the lump while scanning it documents that it is due to fibroglandular tissue (*arrows*). Fibroglandular tissue is a normal component of breast tissue, but merely demonstrating that it exists in the area of a palpable abnormality is insufficient proof that it is the cause of the palpable abnormality. **B:** Palpating while scanning the palpable lump documents that it is due to a simple cyst. Although cysts are not normal, they are common. Merely demonstrating a cyst in the region of the palpable abnormality does not document that the cyst is the cause of the palpable abnormality. **C:** A different patient with a palpable lump. Mammogram showing a small, circumscribed nodule in the area of a palpable lump. **D:** Initial BUS without palpation incorrectly suggested that the palpable lump and mammographic nodule were the same lesion and were the cause of the palpable lump. Palpating while sonographically scanning the lump, however, showed that the mammographic nodule was due to a nonpalpable simple cyst. The palpable lump was due to a shadowing malignant solid lesion immediately adjacent to the simple cyst, which was not visible mammographically.

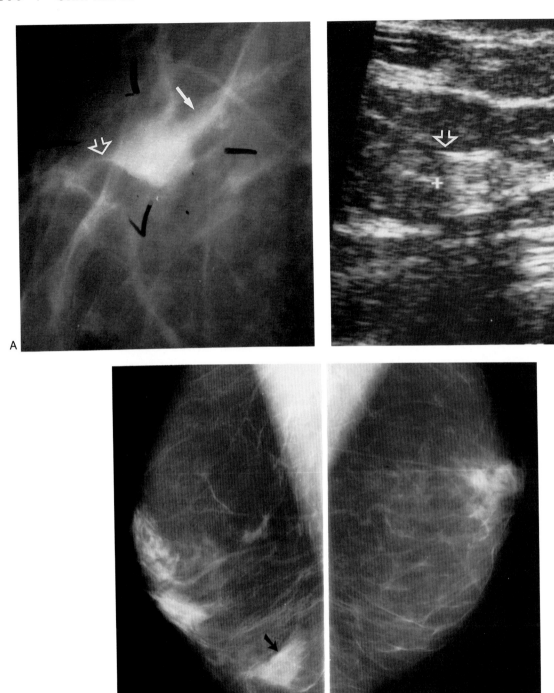

FIG. 10. When the indication for BUS is a mammographic mass, sonography should demonstrate a water density structure in the same location and of the same size and shape as the mammographic lesion. **A:** Patient 1: Mammographic mass that was demonstrable on both craniocaudal (CC) and mediolateral oblique (MLO) views. This magnification CC view shows a broad band of water density tissue extending toward the nipple (*arrow*) and a pointed projection peripherally (*arrowhead*). **B:** Patient 1: Transverse sonographic view shows that the mammographic mass is due to fibroglandular tissue. A broad band of fibroglandular tissue extends toward the nipple (*arrow*), and a narrow point of fibrous tissue extends peripherally (*arrowhead*). The size and location correspond closely to those of the mammographic lesion. This close mammographic-sonographic correlation is critical, since fibroglandular tissue is a normal component of most breasts and merely demonstrating its presence in the general vicinity of the mammographic lesion does not prove that it is the cause of the mammographic density. Correlation is generally better between the CC view of the mammogram and the transverse view of the sonogram than between the MLO mammographic view and the longitudinal or oblique sonographic view. The degree of obliquity on the MLO view is difficult to reproduce sonographically. **C:** Patient 2: A mammographic mass is present inferiorly in the right breast and was visible on both views.

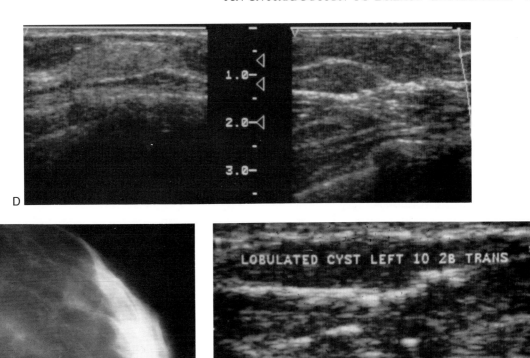

FIG. 10. (*Continued*) **D:** Patient 2: Breast ultrasound split screen views of mirror-image locations inferiorly in both breasts show that the mammographic mass is due to fibroglandular tissues not present in the mirror-image location of the contralateral breast. No water density tissue other than fibroglandular tissue of size and shape similar to the mammographic density was demonstrable in the inferior right breast in the area of the mammographic mass. Split screen views are invaluable in the evaluation of right-to-left focal asymmetric densities or masses. **E:** Patient 3: Craniocaudal projection mammogram shows a lobulated nodule. **F:** Patient 3: Transverse sonogram shows a simple cyst with identically sized and shaped lobules, proving that the cyst is the cause of the mammographic nodule.

densities, and areas of architectural distortion (16). Breast ultrasound can determine whether the water density mammographic abnormality is cystic, solid, or normal fibroglandular tissue. The location and shape of the sonographic findings must correspond to the location and shape of the mammographic finding (47) (Fig. 10). Correlating shape and size between the mammographic craniocaudal view and the sonographic transverse view is usually easiest.

Trying to do more than detect cysts within water density areas on mammograms is highly controversial. Some argue that we should not try to detect solid nodules within water density (8). Others feel that BUS is useful only if a discrete cyst or solid nodule is demonstrated within the area of water density on mammograms (i.e., that a positive BUS is useful) (2,4,8,17,48,49). However, it is clear that the demonstration of a uniformly echogenic focus of fibrous or fibroglandular tissue (water density mammographically) is also useful if its size, shape, and location correspond exactly to the mammographic lesion. Breast cancers may have a rim of echogenicity equal to that of fibroglandular elements, but the centers of these tumors are usually hypoechoic to isoechoic with fat, and virtually none have a central echogenicity equal to that of fibroglandular tissue (22). A focus of increased echogenicity without any internal areas of hypo- or isoechogenicity is fibrous or fibroglandular tissue and not cancer. If, however, there is a lesion of decreased echogenicity within the fibrous tissue, biopsy or follow-up ultrasound is warranted.

Breast ultrasound of focal mammographic asymmetries is also controversial, with some authors recommending against it (6,50). It is true that asymmetries seen only on one view are usually compression artifact and should not be subjected to ultrasound. Focal asymmetries that are clearly present on both views and that remain present but nonspecific on additional mammogram views such as spot compression magnification views, however, should undergo BUS. Careful real-time examination of focal asymmetries frequently shows underlying cysts surrounded by fibrous tissue, obviating the need for further workup or follow-up. In addition, solid nodules can be found within these focal asymmetries far more frequently than these authors suggest.

3. Breast ultrasound can be used in the evaluation of breast secretions when ductography fails or cannot be performed. Ductography is typically the procedure of choice for evaluating abnormal breast secretions but is not always possible or successful. Secretions must be expressible from the nipple at the time of ductogra-phy to allow cannulation of the correct duct. Even in the presence of expressible secretions, cannulation sometimes fails. When ductography is not possible, sonography may be helpful because the offending duct may be obstructed by inspissated secretions (especially when spontaneous secretions stop) and distended with fluid. We scan the breast radially clockwise around the nipple from 12 o'clock, searching for an ectatic duct that is dilated out of proportion to other ducts. After finding such a duct, we position the transducer so that it is parallel to the long axis of the duct. We then search the dilated, fluid-filled duct peripherally for a solid papillary lesion within it—either an intraductal papilloma (90%) or papillary carcinoma (10%) (Figs. 11 and 12). Other less definitive findings, such as a single ectatic duct without an intraductal papillary lesion, may occur. Such ducts usually correspond to the secreting duct. Severe diffuse ductal ectasia may correspond to diffuse papillomatosis. If the lesion requires surgical removal, ductography can be performed with iodinated contrast agent and blue dye on the day of surgery to localize the lesion. If the lesion is visible sonographically, ultrasound-guided needle localization can be performed.

4. Breast ultrasound should be used to follow solid lesions demonstrable only by ultrasound which the patient has elected not to have biopsied. Sonographically and mammographically visible lesions may be followed

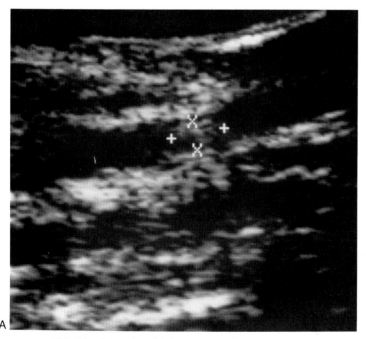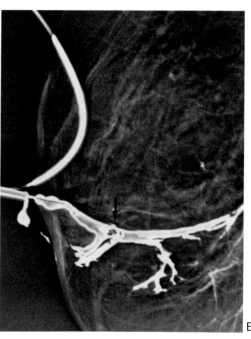

FIG. 11. Cases in which sonography made the initial diagnosis of intraductal papilloma. **A:** Patient 1: Small intraductal papillary lesion demonstrated sonographically because the patient was unable to express secretions on the day of her scheduled ductogram. **B:** Patient 1: Secretions were expressible on the day of surgery. The preoperative ductogram performed for methylene blue dye injection confirmed the location and size of the intraductal lesion, which was proven to be an intraductal papilloma.

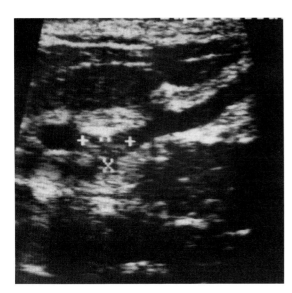

FIG. 12. Intraductal papilloma initially diagnosed by ductography but localized with ultrasound-guided needle localization on the day of surgery because secretions were not expressible preoperatively. The preoperative sonogram shows the expansile papillary lesion within an ectatic fluid-filled duct at 9 o'clock in the left breast.

with mammography, BUS, or both. Alternating mammography and sonography at six-month intervals may also be performed.

5. Use BUS as the primary diagnostic technique for evaluating focal clinical abnormalities during pregnancy, when mammography and radiation exposure are undesirable.

6. Use BUS to evaluate for breast abscess in cases of acute mastitis. Ultrasound may show no abscesses, multiple small abscesses too small to drain, or a dominant abscess (8).

7. Breast ultrasound is ideal for guiding preoperative localization procedures, cyst aspiration, and core needle biopsies (18,20,30,36) (Fig. 13 in this chapter and Figs. 9 in Chapter 12 and 11 in Chapter 13). Obviously, sonographic localization is mandatory for lesions that are visible only by sonography. However, we also prefer sonographic localization for lesions that are both mammographically and sonographically visible. Ultrasound is also mandatory when lesions are visible only on one mammographic view (despite additional mammogram views) unless stereotactic mammography is available (18–20).

Exceptional Indications for Whole-Breast Ultrasound

Although BUS is usually a diagnostic tool and the examination is usually targeted, there are exceptional situations in which unilateral or bilateral whole-breast ultrasound is indicated. Usually, such scans will sup-

plement routine mammography, but on rare occasions they may replace mammography.

1. Whole-breast sonography may supplement mammography in patients who have very dense tissues on mammography and who have a personal or strong family history of breast cancer. Several studies have shown that whole-breast sonography is not helpful in the general population of patients with dense breast tissues (2,4,6,8). However, patients at very high risk for breast cancer, such as those with a positive self-history or a positive family history of breast cancer in mother and sister before age 40 and those with the ataxia-telangiectasia gene (in whom the lifetime risk of cancer is about 50%), should be evaluated with every means of surveillance possible.

2. Whole-breast sonography can supplement mammography and initially evaluate or follow multiple bilateral mammographic and/or follow sonographic abnormalities.

3. Whole-breast sonography can identify a primary neoplasm when metastatic disease of breast origin is suspected and mammography is negative.

4. Whole-breast sonography can replace mammography in patients who have radiation phobia and refuse mammography. Before doing the BUS we will always explain to these patients that mammography is the preferred method of screening for breast cancer and that we recommend mammography over sonography for that purpose. This may be an option chosen more frequently in the future by patients who are homozygous or heterozygous for the ataxia-telangiectasia gene and

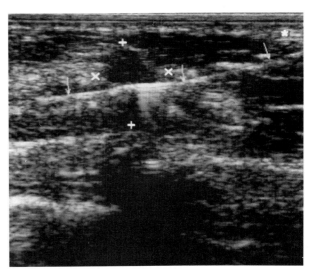

FIG. 13. Ultrasound-guided needle localization of a solid breast nodule after wire and blue dye placement. The braided Hawkins 3 wire is extremely well seen passing through an infiltrating duct carcinoma because of its relatively horizontal course and the high-frequency, near-field, electronically focused linear probe.

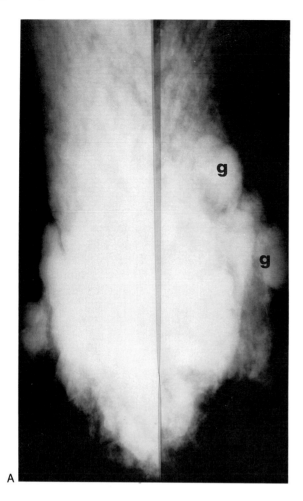

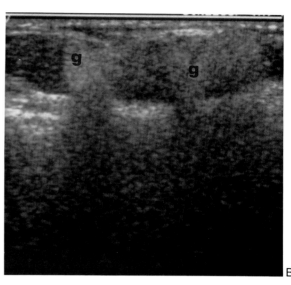

FIG. 14. Free silicone injection into the breasts. **A:** Mammogram shows globules of dense material representing silicone granulomas (*g*) resulting from the injection of free silicone into the breasts. **B:** Sonogram shows foci of intensely echogenic, shadowing material representing the silicone granulomas.

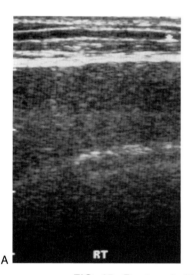

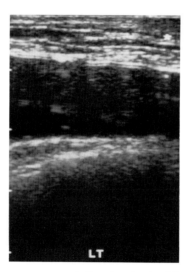

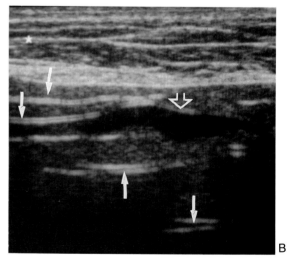

FIG. 15. Ruptured silicone augmentation implant with encapsulated extravasated silicone. **A:** The mammogram showed only a thicker "capsule" around the right implant than around the left. Split screen ultrasound shows echogenic, poorly transmitting encapsulated extravasated silicone on the *right*. The lucent fluid on the *left* is within a normal implant. **B:** Sonographic sections through other portions of the right breast show echogenic parallel lines corresponding to portions of the partially collapsed implant membranes (*arrows*). The lucent area centrally corresponds to unextravasated silicone (*arrowhead*) still within the implant.

in whom the risk of radiation exposure from mammography may be greatly increased.

5. Breast ultrasound has recently become a primary diagnostic tool for diagnosing leaking or ruptured silicone breast implants (51–53). Mammography can readily detect unencapsulated silicone leaks, but it is unable to detect leaks encapsulated within the fibrous pseudocapsule around the implant (Fig. 14). A significant percentage of these silicone implants incite the development of such a "capsule." The free silicone fills the encapsulated space and mammographically "silhouettes" the silicone remaining within the implant and the implant membranes. Breast ultrasound can detect both extracapsular and intracapsular silicone leaks, but the sonographic examination for silicone leaks is usually nontargeted. The extravasated silicone elicits a host response that causes it to become homogeneously echogenic and to transmit sound poorly. This appearance has been called the "snowstorm" appearance. Additionally, convoluted portions of the collapsed implant membranes and silicone within the implant appear as lucent areas within the "snowstorm" (Fig. 15). Breast ultrasound evaluation of implant patients with palpable lumps and mammographic lesions is, of course, similar to targeted examinations in patients without implants (54).

Whole-breast sonographic screening of patients with augmentation implants for cancer is not recommended. The Eklund compression techniques and views have enabled much more complete mammographic evaluation of augmentation implant patients than was previously possible and have made sonographic screening unnecessary (55).

TECHNICAL CONSIDERATIONS

Diagnostic BUS is technically demanding and requires proper equipment and meticulous technique (9,31,38,39,45,55–59).

Equipment Considerations

High-frequency (7 MHz or more) linear electronically focused probes are preferred for BUS. Also, 10 MHz sector probes with built-in stand-off are satisfactory. Because of inherent differences in probe design and software implementation, however, not all 7 to 10 MHz probes are adequate for BUS applications. Technical requirements for BUS are very demanding.

Breast ultrasound requires superb "near-field" spatial resolution. Many breast lesions lie within the superficial centimeter of breast tissue. The depth of breast tissue being evaluated is rarely more than 4 cm in the supine ipsilateral anterior oblique scan position. A probe must have both good axial and good lateral reso-

lution within the zone of interest to have excellent overall spatial resolution (38,44,57–59).

Because axial resolution is inversely proportional to wavelength and wavelengths are shorter for higher frequency probes, axial resolution is better for higher frequency than for lower frequency probes. Furthermore, an acoustic "stand-off" will not help axial resolution, as it does not vary with depth (9,31,38,45).

Lateral resolution (slice thickness) does vary with depth, is more complex, and depends upon several factors: scan line density, fixed elevation plane focal length, and long-axis electronic focusing.

1. A high line density requires a large number of small transducer elements and, in some instances, "half-line" scanning. Most commercial 7 MHz or 7.5 MHz linear probes have adequate line density.

2. Electronic linear probes can be electronically focused only along the long axis of the probe. The focus of the shorter "off-axis" or elevation plane axis of the probe is fixed by an acoustic lens (Fig. 16). The fixed elevation plane focus of the probe must be very superficial, about 1 to 1.5 cm. Unfortunately, most 5 MHz and even some 7 MHz linear probes are focused at 3 to 4 cm, far too deep for adequate breast ultrasound (Fig. 17). If more optimal probes are not available, a stand-off pad or a large amount of jelly used as a stand-off may improve the focusing characteristics of these probes for breast applications.

3. Electronic focusing is available along the long axis of the probe. The probe may be electronically fo-

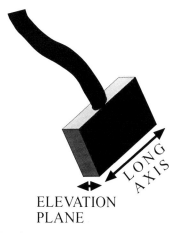

ELEVATION
PLANE

FIG. 16. The linear electronic ultrasound has two axes, the long axis and the elevation plane axis. Individual elements are lined up side by side along the long axis. This enables dynamic electronic focusing in the longitudinal plane. Since there is only a single element in the short (elevation) axis of the probe, electronic focusing is not possible in the elevation plane. Each linear probe has an elevation plane focus that is fixed at one depth. The depth of the elevation plane focus varies from probe to probe, generally (but not always) being more superficial for higher frequency probes.

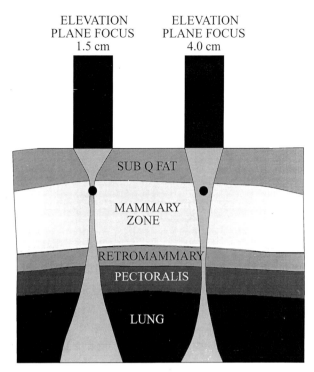

ELEVATION
PLANE FOCUS
1.5 cm

ELEVATION
PLANE FOCUS
4.0 cm

SUB Q FAT

MAMMARY
ZONE

RETROMAMMARY

PECTORALIS

LUNG

FIG. 17. Two linear probes with the same frequency and footprint may have different elevation plane focal lengths. The probe designed as a vascular probe (*right*) may be focused at 4 cm of depth, too deep for BUS in most patients. The beam width throughout the superficial areas of the breast is much wider than for the probe, focused at 1.5 cm. The small mass (*m*) is narrower than the beam width and will be "volume-averaged" with surrounding tissues. This frequently results in mischaracterization of medium- and large-sized cysts because of "filling-in" with echoes from adjacent tissues or even the missing of smaller cysts and solid nodules. The probe optimized for near-field imaging (*left*) is focused at 1.5 cm, ideal for most BUS patients. The small mass is wider than the beam and will be more accurately characterized if centered within the beam.

cused on both receive and transmit. Many commercially available probes have adequate electronic focusing on receive throughout the depth of field. The number and depth of transmit focuses can vary greatly among probes, however. Excellent near-field resolution requires several transmit focusing zones superficial to 2 cm. Most commercially available 5 MHz and even some 7 MHz linear probes do not have enough superficial transmit focal zones for breast ultrasound. Stand-offs can improve the electronic transmit-zone focusing characteristics of these probes for breast ultrasound.

In addition to excellent spatial resolution, breast ultrasound requires superb contrast resolution. Contrast resolution depends upon probe frequency, bandwidth, and other factors. Higher frequencies and broader

bandwidths result in better contrast resolution. Probes with a 7 MHz or higher center frequency and bandwidths of greater than 50% have the best contrast resolution for breast ultrasound (45).

Patient Positioning and Scanning Technique

We place the patient in a supine contralateral posterior oblique position with the ipsilateral arm elevated. The ipsilateral hand is positioned behind the head (Fig. 6 in Chapter 4). Patients with large breasts generally require higher degrees of obliquity than those with small breasts. Evaluation of lateral lesions requires the patient to be positioned in steeper contralateral posterior obliquity. The patient may lie flat on her back for some far-medial lesions. This positioning of the patient accomplishes several things.

1. The breast tissue is thinned to the maximum extent possible, ensuring adequate penetration with the high-frequency beam, which is needed for good spatial and contrast resolution (8).
2. This places most of the tissue planes within the mammary zone of the breast parallel to the transducer face and perpendicular to the ultrasound beam (38,39,56), minimizing reflective and refractive attenuation of the high-frequency beam.
3. The combination of thinned breast tissues and improved specular reflection from normal tissues improves visualization of the needle for localizations, aspirations, and biopsies.
4. The position in which we scan patients is very close to the position in which the patient will be placed for open surgical biopsies.

There are occasional exceptions to this contralateral posterior oblique patient positioning. Palpable abnormalities present only in the upright position generally must be scanned in the upright position. Also, multiple different patient positions may be useful in evaluating suspected fluid-debris levels within complex cysts.

Increasing probe compression pressure thins the tissues being scanned and flattens oblique tissue planes into a plane more perpendicular to the beam. This again results in better penetration and diminished critical angle shadowing from obliquely oriented tissue planes (38). Compression may also be useful in evaluating the compressibility of sonographically identified lesions. Incompressible lesions are more likely to be malignant. Heavy compressive probe pressure should generally be reserved for situations where critical angle shadowing from superficially located Cooper's ligaments prevents the evaluation of deeper tissues. Increased probe pressure may sometimes be counterproductive. Heavy probe pressure for routine scanning can cause pain in patients with tender breasts. It can also continually push true lesions out of the scan plane. Finally, it can alter the depth focal zones in a manner that causes superficial lesions to be missed.

Time-gain compensation curves should be set so that fatty tissues are a medium gray from skin line to pectoralis. Time-gain compensation curves generally are fairly shallow for fatty areas of the breast and steeper for fibroglandular portions of the breast (38). The depth of field should be great enough that the pectoralis muscle, ribs, and pleural line are visible in the deepest part of the field (Fig. 3). All sonographic lesions should be scanned in two orthogonal planes.

Palpable breast abnormalities should be palpated while being scanned. Clearly benign structures such as simple cysts and normal fibroglandular elements may be firm compared to surrounding soft fatty tissues and may, therefore, be palpable as lumps or ridges. Simply demonstrating that cysts or fibroglandular tissues are present in the area of interest is inadequate proof that they are the cause of the palpable abnormality, however (47). Simultaneous palpation and scanning is the only way to prove this conclusively (Fig. 9).

A wide area around the suspected location of a mammographic lesion must sometimes be scanned. Some nodules may move several centimeters when compressed for mammography. This is especially true of lesions seen on routine oblique mammogram views, where movement is in the craniocaudal axis. Mammographic densities that may appear to be in the upper half of the breast on oblique views may actually lie straight laterally or even slightly inferiorly at the time of ultrasound. Lesions that are near 3 o'clock or 9 o'clock tend to move up or down the most with compression. If we do not immediately identify the cause of a mammographic density where we suspect it should be from mammographic examination, we scan a 90° wedge of tissue centered on the area of suspicion. Only when we have scanned a wide enough area to encompass the possible range of motion due to compression can we be sure that we have not simply geographically missed a lesion.

Palpable nodules that are very small and characterized as pea or BB sized are usually very near the skin. Even with optimal high-frequency, near-field probes, these lesions may be too close to the skin to be resolved or appropriated characterized without the use of a stand-off. Less optimally focused 5 MHz probes may require a stand-off of 1 to 3 cm. More ideally configured 7 or 7.5 MHz probes may require only a jelly stand-off of a few extra millimeters. Very small lesions near the skin may be either completely missed due to their location superficial to the focal planes of the probe or mischaracterized. Cysts may appear solid because of side-lobe artifacts, which are most pronounced in the

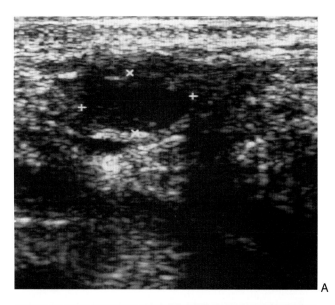

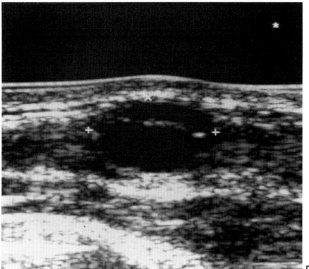

FIG. 18. Near-field artifact leads to mischaracterization of a septate simple cyst. **A:** Near-field artifact causes the wall of this superficial cyst to appear thickened, requiring classification as a complex cyst. **B:** Scanning through a 1-cm-thick standoff pad "clears" the near-field artifact from the cyst and shows it to have only a thin septum anteriorly and no wall thickening.

very near field. Stand-offs will improve these situations (38,49,57–59) (Fig. 18).

CONCLUSION

Breast ultrasound is a valuable tool in breast diagnosis. Most examinations are targeted at nonspecific clinical or mammographic abnormalities. Breast ultrasound should not be used, however, to evaluate a suspicious cluster of microcalcifications. Such clusters may warrant biopsy regardless of the sonographic findings, making sonographic evaluation superfluous. Breast ultrasound, of course, is the method of choice for determining whether an abnormality is cystic or solid. It can also detect normal fibrous elements in the breast, which are firmer to palpation and radiographically denser than are surrounding fatty tissues. Breast ultrasound can prevent unnecessary biopsy by demonstrating that a palpable abnormality or mammographic density is merely due to a simple cyst or a localized collection of fibrous tissues. Since both cysts and fibrous tissues are common and/or normal components of the breast, great care must be taken to make sure that they actually correspond to the clinical or mammographic abnormality at which BUS was targeted.

Discrete palpable lumps and mammographic nodules shown to be solid can be biopsied immediately, avoiding six-month delays in diagnosis and avoiding the associated anxiety of waiting for a definitive diagnosis. Additionally, aggressive BUS of subtle asymmetric mammographic densities or palpable abnormalities that alone are too minimal to warrant biopsy also leads to the detection of additional solid nodules.

Breast ultrasound can also be used for very specific applications, such as the detection of intraductal papillary lesions in patients with abnormal breast secretions when galactography is not possible. It is the method of choice for detecting leaking silicone implants.

Breast ultrasound can be used in a nontargeted fashion to supplement mammography in patients with very dense breast tissues and very strong family or self-histories or to find a mammographically undetected primary tumor in some patients with metastatic breast cancer.

Finally, BUS is superb at guiding needle localization, aspiration, or core biopsy of sonographically visible lesions.

REFERENCES

1. Moskowitz M. Screening is not diagnosis. *Radiology* 1979;133: 265–268.
2. Sickles EA, Filly RA, Callen PW. Breast cancer detection with sonomammography and mammography: comparison using state-of-the-art equipment. *AJR Am J Roentgenol* 1983;140:843–845.
3. ACR Committee on Breast Imaging. *Policy statement on sonography for the detection and diagnosis of breast disease*, 1984.
4. Kopans DB, Meyer JE, Lindfors KK. Whole-breast ultrasound imaging: four year follow-up. *Radiology* 1985;157:505–507.
5. Dempsey PJ, Moskowitz M. Is there a role for breast sonography? *Clin Diagn Ultrasound* 1987;20:17–36.
6. Bassett LW, Kimme-Smith C, Sutherland LK, et al. Automated and hand-held breast ultrasound: effect on patient management. *Radiology* 1987;165:103–108.
7. Jackson VP. Sonography of malignant breast disease. *Semin Ultrasound CT MR* 1989;10(2):119–131.
8. Jackson VP. The role of ultrasound in breast imaging. *Radiology* 1990;177:305–311.
9. Dempsey PJ. The importance of resolution in the clinical application of the breast sonography. *Ultrasound Med Biol* 1988; 14(1):43–48.
10. Croll J, Kotevich J, Tabretet M. The diagnosis of benign disease and the exclusion of malignancy in patients with breast symptoms. *Semin Ultrasound CT MR* [*in press*].
11. Cole-Beuglet C, Soriano RZ, Kurtz AB, Goldberg BB. Ultrasound analysis of 104 primary breast carcinomas classified according to histopathologic type. *Radiology* 1983;147:191–196.
12. Jellins J, Reeve TS, Croll J, Kossoff G. Results of breast echographic examinations in Sydney, Australia, 1972–1979. *Semin Ultrasound CT MR* 1982;3:58–62.
13. Egan RL, Egan KL. Detection of breast carcinoma: comparison of automated water-path whole-breast sonography, mammography, and physical examination. *AJR Am J Roentgenol* 1984;143: 493–497.
14. Smallwood JA, Guyer P, Dewbury K, et al. The accuracy of ultrasound in the diagnosis of breast disease. *Ann R Coll Surg Engl* 1986;68:19–22.
15. Van Dam PA, Van Goethem MLA, Kersschot E, et al. Palpable solid breast masses: retrospective single and multimodality evaluation of 201 lesions. *Radiology* 1988;166:435–439.
16. Dempsey PJ. Breast sonography: historical perspective, clinical application, and image interpretation. *Ultrasound Q* 1988;6: 69–90.
17. Basset LW, Kimme-Smith C. Breast sonography. *AJR Am J Roentgenol* 1991;156:449–455.
18. D'Orsi CJ, Mendelson EB. Interventional breast ultrasonography. *Semin Ultrasound CT MR* 1989;10:132–138.
19. Kopans DB, Meyer JE, Lindfors KK, et al. Breast sonography to guide cyst aspiration and wire localization of occult solid lesions. *AJR Am J Roentgenol* 1984;143:489–492.
20. Laing FC, Jeffrey RB, Minagi H. Ultrasound localization of occult breast lesions. *Radiology* 1984;151:795–796.
21. Leucht, W. Foreword. In: *Teaching atlas of breast ultrasound*. New York: Thieme; 1984.
22. Kobayashi T. Diagnostic ultrasound in breast cancer: analysis of retrotumorous echo patterns correlated with sonic attenuation by cancerous connective tissue. *J Clin Ultrasound* 1979;7: 471–479.
23. Kopans DB. What is a useful adjunct to mammography? *Radiology* 1986;161:560–561.
24. Fornage BD. Breast ultrasound wins slow acceptance in USA. *Diagn Imaging* 1990;12(10):194.
25. Texidor HS, Kazam E. Combined mammographic-sonographic evaluation of breast masses. *AJR Am J Roentgenol* 1977;128: 409–417.
26. Jellins J, Kossoff G, Reeve TS, Barraclough BH. Detection and classification of liquid-filled masses in the breast by gray-scale echography. *Radiology* l975;125:205–212.
27. Maturo VG, Zusmer NR, Gilson AJ, Bear B. Ultrasonic appearance of mammary carcinoma with a dedicated whole-breast scanner. *Radiology* 1982;142:713–718.
28. Kalisher L. Factors influencing false negative rates in xeromammography. *Radiology* 1979;133:297–301.
29. Martin J, Moskowitz M, Milbrath JR. Breast cancers missed by mammography. *AJR Am J Roentgenol* 1979;132:737–739.
30. Fornage BD, Faroux MJ, Simatos A. Breast masses: ultrasound-guided fine-needle aspiration biopsy. *Radiology* 1987;162: 409–414.
31. Parker SH, Lovin, Jobe WE, Luethke JM, Hopper KD, Yakes WF, Burke BJ. Stereotactic breast biopsy with a biopsy gun. *Radiology* 1990;176:741–747.
32. Parker SH, Lovin JD, Jobe WE, Burke BJ, Hopper KD, Yakes WF. Nonpalpable breast lesions: stereotactic automated large-core biopsies. *Radiology* 1991;180:403–407.
33. Parker SH, Jobe WE. Large-core breast biopsy offers reliable diagnosis. *Diagn Imaging* 1990;12(10):90–97.
34. Rizzatto G, Solbiati L, Croce F, Derchi LE. Aspiration biopsy of superficial lesions: ultrasonic guidance with a linear-array probe. *AJR Am J Roentgenol* 1987;148:623–625.
35. Grant EG, Richardson JD, Smirniotopoulos JG, Jacobs NM. Fine-needle biopsy directed by real-time sonography: technique and accuracy. *AJR Am J Roentgenol* 1983;141:29–32.
36. Ueno E, Aiyoshhi Y, Imamura A, et al. Ultrasonographically guided biopsy of nonpalpable lesions of the breast by the spot method. *Surg Gynecol Obstet* 1990;170:153–155.

37. Harper AP, Kelly-Frye E. Ultrasound visualization of the breast in symptomatic patients. *Radiology* 1980;137:465–467.
38. Bassett LW, Kimme-Smith C. Breast sonography: technique, equipment, and normal anatomy. *Semin Ultrasound CT MR* 1989;10(2):82–89.
39. Schenck CD, Lehman DA. Sonographic anatomy of the breast. *Semin Ultrasound* 1982;3:13–33.
40. Barth V. *Atlas of diseases of the breast*. Chicago: Year Book; 1979.
41. Vorherr H. *The breast: morphology, physiology, and lactation*. New York: Academic Press; Harcourt, Brace, Jovanovich; 1974.
42. Ingleby H, Gershon-Cohen J. *Comparative anatomy, pathology, and roentgenology of the breast*. Chatam, Great Britain: University of Pennsylvania Press; W & J Mackay; 1960.
43. Rogers K, Coup AJ. *Surgical pathology of the breast*. Boston: Wright Publishers, 1990.
44. Adler DD. Ultrasound of benign breast conditions. *Semin Ultrasound CT MR* 1989;10:106–118.
45. Jackson VP, Kelly-Fry E, Rothschild PA, et al. Automated breast sonography using a 7.5 mHz PVDF transducer: preliminary clinical evaluation. *Radiology* 1986;159:679–684.
46. Kimme-Smith C, Bassett LW, Gold RH. High frequency breast ultrasound: hand-held versus screening. *J Ultrasound Med* 1988;7:77–81.
47. Feig SA. The role of ultrasound in a breast imaging center. *Semin Ultrasound CT MR* 1989;10:90–105.
48. Hilton SW, Leoplold GR, Olson LK, et al. Real-time breast sonography: application in 300 consecutive patients. *AJR Am J Roentgenol* 1986;147:479–486.
49. Sickles EA, Filly RA, Callen PW. Benign breast lesions: ultrasound detection and diagnosis. *Radiology* 1984;151:467–470.
50. Kopans DB, Swann CA, White G, et al. Asymmetric breast tissue. *Radiology* 1989;171:639–643.
51. Levine RA, Collins TL. Definitive diagnosis of breast implant rupture by ultrasonography. *Plast Reconstr Surg* 1991;87:1126–1128.
52. Herzog P. Silicone granulomas: detection by ultrasonography [Letter]. *Plast Reconstr Surg* 1989;84:856.
53. Anderson B, Hawtof D, Alani H, Kapetansky D. The diagnosis of ruptured breast implants. *Plast Reconstr Surg* 1989;84:903.
54. Leibman JA, Kruse B. Breast cancer: mammographic and sonographic findings after enhancement mammoplasty. *Radiology* 1990;174:195–198.
55. Eklund GW, Busby RC, Miller SH, Job JS. Improved imaging of the augmented breast. *AJR Am J Roentgenol* 1988;151:469–473.
56. Kossoff G, Jellins J. The physics of breast echography. *Semin Ultrasound* 1982;3:5–12.
57. Rubin E, Miller VE, Berland LL, et al. Hand-held real-time breast sonography. *AJR Am J Roentgenol* 1985;14:623–629.
58. Kimme-Smith C, Hansen M, Bassett LW, et al. Ultrasound mammography effects of focal zone placement. *Radiographics* 1985;5:955–970.
59. Kimme-Smith C, Rothschild PA, Bassett LW, et al. Ultrasound artifacts affect the diagnosis of breast masses. *Ultrasound Med Biol* 1988;14[Suppl 1]:103–210.

Percutaneous Breast Biopsy, edited by
Steve H. Parker and William E. Jobe.
Raven Press, Ltd., New York © 1993.

CHAPTER 11

The Ultrasound of Breast Pathology

A. Thomas Stavros and Mark A. Dennis

Sonographically identified breast lesions can be classified as either cystic or solid. As in other organs, cystic lesions can be classified as simple or complex cysts. There are several different types of complex cystic lesions that differ in their significance. Solid lesions can also be classified by sonographic characteristics into various risk categories.

THE SONOGRAPHY OF CYSTIC BREAST LESIONS

The sonographic characteristics of simple cysts in the breast are the same as those of simple cysts in other organs. They are anechoic; have smooth, well-circumscribed margins; have enhanced through-transmission deep to them; and have thin edge shadows (Fig. 1). If a cystic lesion meets all of these strict sonographic criteria, it is a simple cyst (1–4). Enhanced through-transmission may be difficult to demonstrate for very small cysts and those near the chest wall, however. Sometimes special tangential or coronal views are necessary to demonstrate enhanced through-transmission in cysts near the chest wall (3,5). Sometimes it is demonstrable only on one view (3).

Floating cholesterol crystals may develop in the internal fluid of some chronic cysts. These crystals may cause a low-level echogenicity within the cysts that can make them appear solid (Fig. 2A). It is possible to create a visible swirling and streaming of these crystals within the cyst with the energy of the ultrasound beam by centering the transducer directly over the cyst, holding it very still, adjusting the transmit focus to the center of the cyst, and turning up the power or output of the probe. The energy contained within the sonographic beam is sufficient to push the crystals down through the center of the cyst along the ultrasound beam. Demonstration of this streaming motion confirms the presence of only crystalline material within the cyst and indicates that it is a simple cystic lesion (Fig. 2B). Cysts with low-level internal echoes that cannot be made to move usually contain more viscous fluid with heavier particulate matter and are more likely to contain pus or blood. If the apparent particles cannot be made to move with the energy of the ultrasound beam, aspiration should be performed (Fig. 2C).

Simple breast cysts have virtually no possibility of being malignant and if asymptomatic do not require further diagnostic testing, aspiration, biopsy, or follow-up imaging (3,4,6). Simple cysts are very common and essentially are variants of normal. Merely demonstrating a simple cyst does not prove that it is the cause of the clinical problem or mammographic density. Palpation during scanning is required to prove that a cyst is the cause of a lump. Correlation of location, size, and shape is necessary to prove that the cyst is the cause of the mammographic abnormality (7). Showing that the mammographic abnormality disappears on repeat mammograms after aspiration can also prove that the cyst was the cause of the density. If these clinical and/or mammographic correlations do not conclusively prove that the cyst is the cause of the abnormality for which the sonogram was performed, the areas around the cyst must be carefully interrogated for subtle solid lesions. Although cancers within simple cysts rarely occur, occasional cancers reside immediately adjacent to simple cysts (Fig. 9 in Chapter 10). In such cases a simple cyst may be a sentinel that indicates a focal area

A.T. Stavros and M.A. Dennis: Radiology Imaging Associates, Breast Diagnostic and Counseling Centre, Englewood, Colorado 80111.

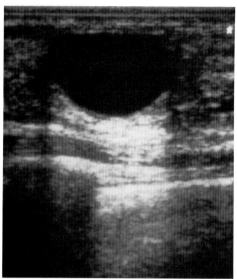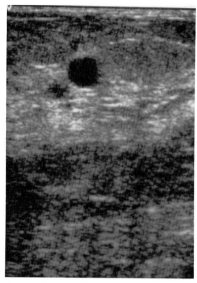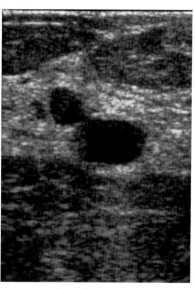

A,B

C

FIG. 1. Simple breast cysts. **A:** This moderate size cyst is completely sonolucent and has enhanced through-transmission, thin edge shadows (the tadpole sign), and a well-circumscribed thin echogenic wall. **B:** This small breast cyst is sonolucent and has thin edge shadows and a well-circumscribed echogenic rim. Enhanced through-transmission is less prominent for smaller cysts and may be difficult to demonstrate for very small cysts. **C:** A simple breast cyst deep to fibroglandular elements shows less-well-defined walls and some internal scatter echoes. Fibroglandular elements superficial to a cyst scatter the ultrasound beam and create artifact, which makes it more difficult to characterize the cyst accurately. It may be helpful to scan with a lower frequency probe in such cases. A complex "thick-walled" cyst is immediately adjacent and superficial to the simple cyst.

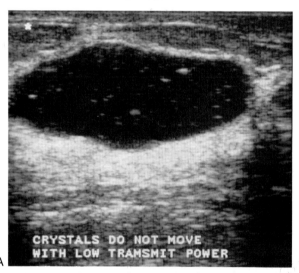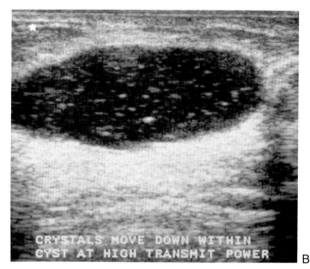

CRYSTALS DO NOT MOVE
WITH LOW TRAMSMIT POWER

A

CRYSTALS MOVE DOWN WITHIN
CYST AT HIGH TRANSMIT POWER

B

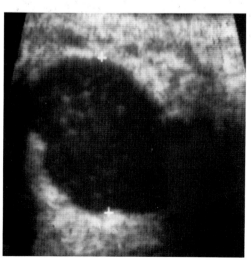

C

FIG. 2. Complex cysts with diffuse low-level internal echoes. **A:** Patient 1: Breast cyst with low-level internal echoes due to cholesterol crystals at normal power settings. The echoes do not move. The cyst could be mistaken for a solid lesion or an infected or hemorrhagic cyst. With higher probe frequencies and a narrower beam width, cholesterol crystals can be demonstrated within chronic simple cysts. **B:** Patient 1: The cholesterol crystals are pushed downward centrally by the beam energy at full power settings and swirl back up peripherally. The swirling motion indicates that the lesion is not solid and, furthermore, that this is a simple cyst with cholesterol crystals. We have not seen such swirling movement with heavier blood or pus elements in hemorrhagic or infected cysts. **C:** Patient 2: Infected, reaccumulated cyst postaspiration. There are diffuse low-level but more heterogeneous echoes within the cyst, and the walls appear thickened and less well defined. The echoes within the cyst could not be made to move with percussion or with the energy of the ultrasound beam.

of hyperstimulation. In such a stimulated milieu, the development of an associated cancer may theoretically be more likely.

There are several different categories of complex cysts. Complex breast cysts usually do not indicate the same increased risk of malignancy that is indicated by complex cysts of other organs (such as the kidneys). For some categories of complex cysts, however, the risk of malignancy may be significantly higher than it is for a simple cyst.

Most cysts containing low-level homogeneous echoes are simple cysts with floating cholesterol crystals, as described above. Complex cysts have more heterogeneous internal echoes that cannot be made to stream. Another manifestation of such a complex cyst may be a gravity-dependent fluid-debris level within the lesion (Fig. 3). Whether there are echoes scattered throughout the cyst or layered in a fluid-debris level may merely depend upon how long the patient has been in one position. Such cysts may be infected or hemorrhagic (4,8). There is probably enough difference in risk between this type of complex cyst and typical simple cysts to justify aspiration and possible core biopsy of portions of the wall, especially if there are signs of infection or inflammation.

Septated cysts represent a heterogeneous group. Cysts that have a single thin septum within them should be treated like simple cysts (8) (Fig. 4A). These septa probably merely represent infolding of the thin cyst wall, a bend in a severely ectatic duct, or walls between adjacent cysts. Cysts with thick internal septa have a higher likelihood of being malignant, however, and should be aspirated/biopsied (Fig. 4B). Complex cysts containing numerous thin septa most frequently represent clusters of multiple smaller simple cysts (8) (Fig. 5). These probably arise as a cluster of hyperplastic ectatic ducts and/or ductolobular complexes (Fig. 6). The clinical significance of such clustered cysts is probably little different from that of simple cysts (8). It may, however, be difficult to be absolutely certain that such a complex cyst is merely a cluster of smaller simple cysts or ectatic ducts and not a very hypoechoic solid nodule with low-level internal echoes. In such cases, aspiration should be attempted. Some complex cysts that are composed of numerous simple cysts can be aspirated because the cysts communicate with each other, but others cannot be aspirated because the cysts do not communicate with each other and each component cyst has too little fluid. Such lesions should be treated as if they were solid. We now try to schedule patients with isolated lesions of this type for ultrasound-guided aspiration with core biopsy to follow if the lesion cannot be completely aspirated. Some patients may have many of these indeterminate lesions bilaterally. In such cases aspiration and biopsy of every lesion may be impractical, and only the largest and most worrisome lesion(s) on each side should be investigated, provided that the patient is followed with mam-

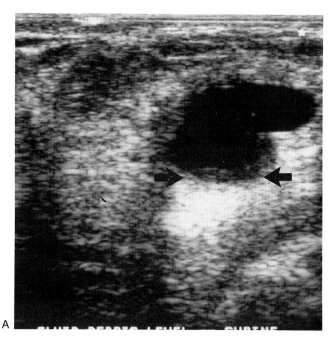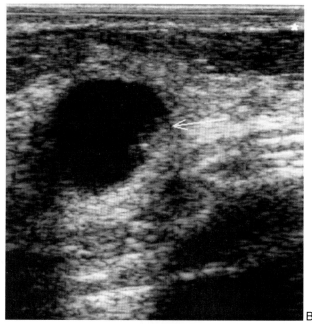

FIG. 3. Fluid-debris level within a complex breast cyst. **A:** Transverse view of a fluid-debris level (*arrowheads*) with the patient in the supine position. **B:** The fluid-debris level has shifted toward the left wall of the cyst with the patient in the left lateral decubitus position; this shift is similar to that of sludge within the gallbladder. The postaspiration view showed the complex cyst completely drained. Aspiration yielded bloody fluid with benign cytologic findings. Excisional biopsy revealed a benign but hemorrhagic cyst.

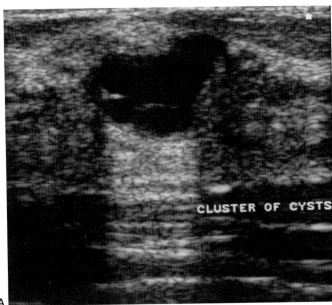
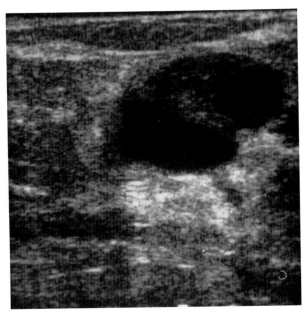

FIG. 4. Lobulated, septate breast cyst. **A:** The cyst has all of the benign characteristics except for the thin internal septa. These may represent the walls between multiple clustered simple cysts or vessels or nerves indenting the cyst walls. The risk of malignancy is little different from that of a single simple cyst. **B:** This complex cyst has a very thick internal septum. The implications are very different from those of thin septa. This was an intracystic carcinoma in a pregnant patient under 30 years of age.

mography and ultrasound in six months. Alternatively, aspiration and biopsy may be avoided altogether by following all lesions with mammography and sonography in six months.

Thick-walled cysts represent another category of

complex cysts. There are two subcategories of these lesions: those with concave thickening of the wall (Fig. 7) and those with convex thickening of the wall or a mural nodule (Fig. 8). The latter subcategory is much more likely to represent an intracystic papilloma or

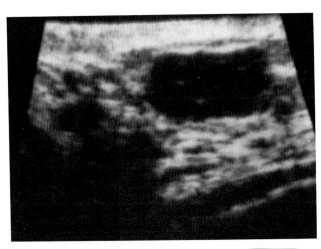

FIG. 5. Complex cyst due to a cluster of very small simple cysts. Only the anterior and posterior walls of the individual small, simple cysts are demonstrable. Lateral walls are poorly demonstrated because of critical angle reflection and refraction. The risk of malignancy is similar to that of simple cysts and cysts with thin internal septations. When the individual cysts are very small (1 to 2 mm), it can be impossible to determine whether such lesions are complex cystic or solid. Such lesions should be assumed to be solid until proven otherwise.

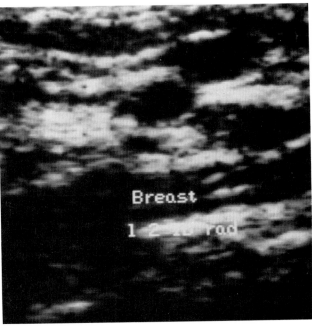

FIG. 6. Clusters of cystically dilated ductules. Individually dilated ductules probably represent the earliest form of the clustered cysts noted in Fig. 5.

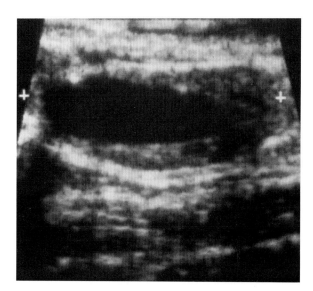

FIG. 7. Complex cyst with a concave, thickened wall. The wall around the right side of the cyst is grossly thickened. The thickening is concave inward. Although the appearance is worrisome and aspiration and/or biopsy is recommended, all nonseptate complex cysts with concave, thickened outer walls that we have biopsied have been benign.

carcinoma than is the former (8–13). Complex cysts with concave wall thickening are very unlikely to represent cancer, but the risks of all thick-walled complex cysts are greater than for any of the other complex cystic lesions described above (8). Regardless of the specific characteristics, however, ultrasound-guided cyst aspiration and core biopsy of the thickened wall or mural nodule or excisional biopsy should be done.

THE SONOGRAPHY OF SOLID BREAST LESIONS

Because an absolute benign vs. malignant distinction is not possible with ultrasound alone, most solid breast nodules will be biopsied regardless of their sonographic characteristics (1,3,14–25). Despite this, it is valuable to use sonographic characteristics to determine the likelihood of malignancy because it may be helpful to both clinicians and the patient to have some idea of risk before biopsy. Relatively high probabilities of malignancy may alter the patient's decision about whether and when to undergo biopsy. A high probability of malignancy may also alter the surgeon's choice of biopsy type. In patients with multiple solid lesions bilaterally, characterization of the lesions may aid in selecting which lesions to biopsy. A patient who is told only that she has a solid nodule that may be malignant and that should be biopsied is usually emotionally distraught. Although it is perfectly appropriate to be worried about an impending and unavoidable biopsy, it can be reassuring to patients to be informed that the chances of malignancy are less than 5%. Knowing that a solid nodule has a low risk of malignancy can also affect the patient's choice of type of biopsy. Patients with a solid nodule who are informed that it has a low risk of malignancy may be more likely to choose core biopsy over excisional biopsy. This is especially true if they have previously had multiple open biopsies of benign lesions.

The following characteristics of solid breast lesions can be evaluated: echogenicity, internal texture, margins, sound transmission, and shape. Each nodule can then be classified into one of three groups:

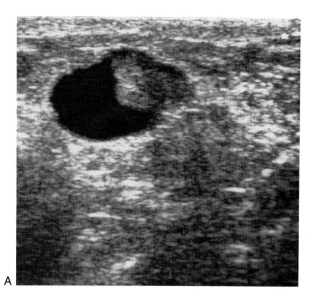

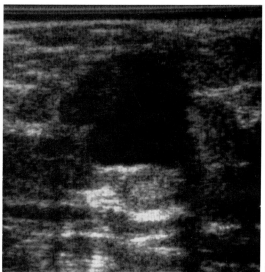

A   B

FIG. 8. Complex cyst with inward convexity of a thickened wall or a mural nodule. **A:** Patient 1: Another intracystic papilloma with a mural nodule. **B:** Patient 2: An intracystic carcinoma that is sonographically indistinguishable from intracystic papilloma. Aggressive aspiration and core biopsy or excisional biopsy is recommended for all complex cysts with mural nodules.

- solid, probably malignant; 50% or greater chance of malignancy
- solid, atypical; 5% to 49% chance of malignancy;
- solid probably benign, less than 5% chance of malignancy.

THE SONOGRAPHIC CHARACTERISTICS ASSOCIATED WITH MALIGNANCY

Findings with a high probability of association with carcinoma include

- marked hypoechogenicity (Fig. 9);
- angular margins (Fig. 10);
- a thick, echogenic rim with perpendicular echoes (Fig. 11);
- shadowing (Fig. 12);
- calcifications (Fig. 13); and
- an anteroposterior dimension greater than the transverse dimension (Fig. 14).

Most infiltrating breast carcinomas are markedly hypoechoic and quite conspicuous, whether they are surrounded by hyperechoic fibrous tissues or isoechoic fatty tissues (18,26–30) (Fig. 9). A smaller percentage of cancers is isoechoic or only mildly hypoechoic with respect to fat, and these are less conspicuous, especially when surrounded by fat. Markedly hypoechoic solid nodules are more likely to be grossly infiltrating carcinomas, whereas mildly hypoechoic lesions are more likely to be DCIS or medullary or colloid carci-

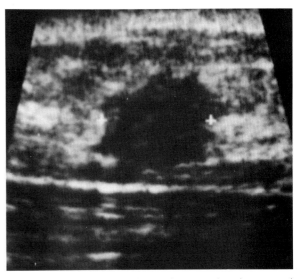

FIG. 10. Infiltrating ductal carcinoma showing angular margins. These angles may be acute, 90°, or obtuse. Fibroadenomas and even DCIS tend to have rounded rather than angular margins.

noma (18,26,27,31–33). (Many fibroadenomas are also mildly hypoechoic.)

Infiltrating cancers frequently have irregular and angular margins. The border of the hypoechoic portion of the lesion has corners and makes abrupt turns and angles (18,26–30) (Fig. 10). Angular margins are much more frequently seen with grossly infiltrating cancers than with DCIS, medullary carcinoma, or colloid carcinoma (18,26,31,33). One author stated, however, that most medullary carcinomas are sonographically spiculated (27). Benign solid nodules rarely have angular margins. Fibroadenomas have either smooth ovoid or gently lobulated surfaces (8,23,30).

Thick echogenic rims that have echoes oriented perpendicular to the surface of the nodule (spiculation) are usually associated with scirrhous infiltrating cancers (28,31,34) (Fig. 11). If surrounded by fat, these lesions correspond to the classic cancer on mammography. If the lesion is surrounded by fibrous tissue and without clustered calcifications, however, the sonogram may be more definitive than is mammography. Noninvasive intraductal carcinomas and fibroadenomas have a thin echogenic rim (pseudocapsule) with echoes oriented parallel to the surface of the lesion.

Some cancers transmit sound poorly and cast an acoustic shadow deep to various portions of the nodule (Fig. 12). The propensity of a nodule to shadow depends not only on the lesion but also on the probe configuration. Shadowing is more common with 10 MHz probes than with lower frequency probes and is more common with sector probes than with the linear probes that are now in use. Shadowing is more likely to be associated with fibrous elements in grossly infil-

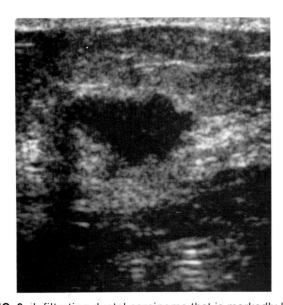

FIG. 9. Infiltrating ductal carcinoma that is markedly hypoechoic with respect to the surrounding mammary fat. Fibroadenomas tend to be only mildly hypoechoic or isoechoic with mammary fat, whereas the majority of infiltrating cancers are very hypoechoic.

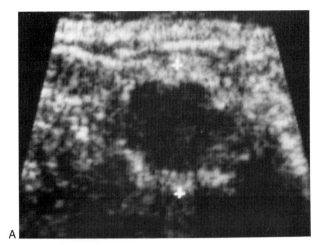
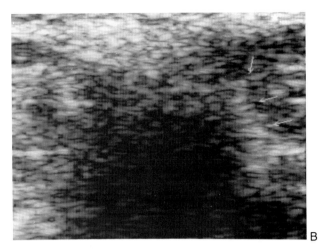

A   B

FIG. 11. Infiltrating ductal carcinomas with thick echogenic rims. **A:** Patient 1: Ill-defined thick echogenic rim, which should be contrasted with the well-circumscribed thin echogenic pseudocapsule seen in the fibroadenomas in Fig. 15. This lesion is also markedly hypoechoic and transmits sound poorly. **B:** Patient 2: Thick echogenic rim with echoes that are perpendicular to the surface of the nodule. The lesion is also markedly hypoechoic and has angular margins.

trating cancers than with DCIS or tumors with only microscopic infiltration (18,19,26,27,30,35,36). Most fibroadenomas have thin edge shadows similar to those of a simple cyst (15,18,19,26,27,30,35–37).

Many microcalcifications are not visible sonographically, and ultrasound should not be used to screen for calcifications or to decide whether to biopsy an isolated cluster of calcifications (1,28,38–42). Calcifications that are visible are usually within breast nodules, which are far more likely to be associated with malignant than with benign lesions (26,31,38) (Fig. 13). This is because

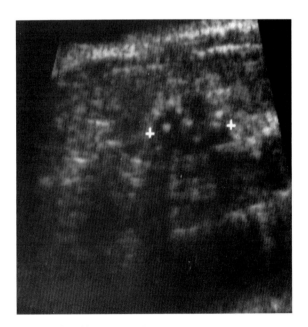

FIG. 13. Calcifications within breast carcinoma. Calcifications within cancers are small, bright echogenicities visible sonographically because they lie within a background of marked hypoechogenicity. Although most breast calcifications are not visible sonographically, those that are sonographically demonstrable are much more likely to be malignant. Most sonographically visible malignant calcifications are too small to shadow, however. Calcifications may be seen sonographically within infiltrating ductal carcinoma or DCIS. Although the positive predictive value of such sonographically visible calcifications is high, the sensitivity of BUS for such calcifications is relatively low compared to that of mammography. Breast ultrasound should not be used to evaluate worrisome calcifications on mammograms.

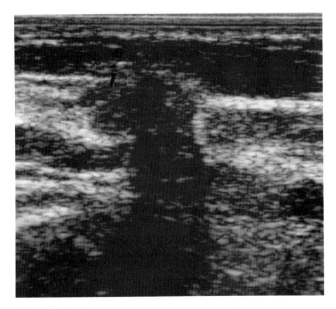

FIG. 12. Infiltrating ductal carcinoma that shadows intensely and is markedly hypoechoic. Most cancers that shadow intensely are also markedly hypoechoic. This lesion also demonstrates angular margins.

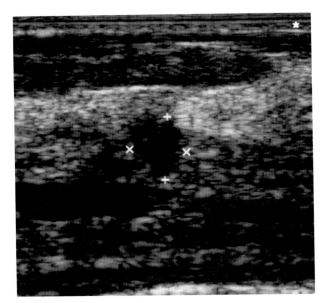

FIG. 14. Infiltrating ductal carcinoma that has a greater depth dimension than transverse dimension. In the supine position, the normal tissue planes of the breast are horizontal. Lesions that are "taller" than they are wide are growing across tissue planes rather than within them, a malignant characteristic. The positive predictive value of such a finding is high, but the sensitivity is low. This lesion also demonstrates marked hypoechogenicity, angular margins, and a poorly defined thick echogenic rim.

the markedly hyperechoic bright white calcifications are more conspicuous within the markedly hypoechoic cancers than they are within more hyperechoic normal and benign pathologic tissues (26).

Nodules that are taller than they are wide are more likely to be malignant (29,32,43–45). Such a shape indicates growth of the nodule across normal tissue planes, which are parallel to the chest wall and skin line (Fig. 14). Benign lesions, such as fibroadenomas, grow horizontally within the normal tissue planes and are wider than they are tall. Although many cancers are not larger in the anteroposterior (AP) dimension than in the transverse dimension (low sensitivity), the presence of a nodule with such a shape strongly favors malignancy (high positive predictive value) (43).

ATYPICAL SONOGRAPHIC CHARACTERISTICS

Atypical sonographic characteristics have more than a 5% but less than a 50% association with malignancy. Atypical findings include

– lobulation (Figs. 15 and 16),
– heterogeneous echotexture (Figs. 15 and 16),
– duct extension (Fig. 17), and
– branch pattern (Fig. 17).

Lobulation and heterogeneity usually occur together (33). Although smaller fibroadenomas are typically

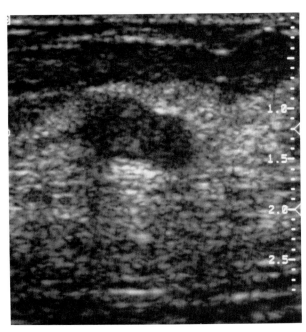

FIG. 15. Lobulation and internal textural heterogeneity. This large fibroadenoma has two gentle lobules and a homogeneous internal texture. Lobulation and heterogeneity are mildly atypical features, since they are associated with a mildly increased chance of malignancy. The vast majority of gently lobulated, heterogeneous solid breast masses are fibroadenomas, however. Two or three gentle lobules should be distinguished, however, from microlobules, as noted in Fig. 16.

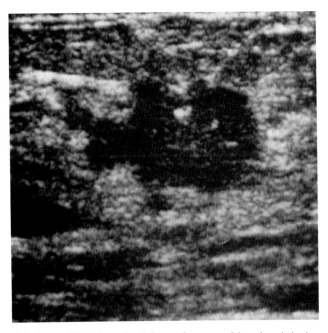

FIG. 16. Infiltrating ductal carcinoma with microlobulation and heterogeneous texture. The lobules are smaller and more numerous than the two or three gentle lobules that are seen with larger fibroadenomas. These microlobules actually represent tumor within individual ductal components. Such microlobulated masses are analogous to the "knobby carcinomas" described in the early literature of mammography. This carcinoma also demonstrates calcifications.

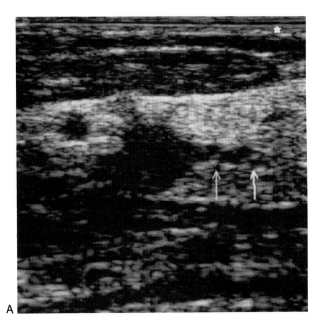
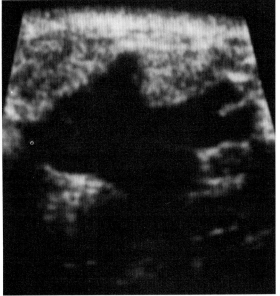

A B

FIG. 17. Duct extension and branch pattern demonstrated by scanning in the radial plane. **A:** Patient 1: Radial scan shows extension of this mass through a duct toward the nipple (*arrows*). This mass also demonstrates marked hypoechogenicity and spiculation. **B:** Patient 2: Radial scan of another carcinoma shows extension of tumor from the main part of the mass peripherally (away from the nipple, which is off the left side of the image) into several ducts. Standard longitudinal and transverse scans showed only lobulation and heterogeneity, which have a much lower positive predictive value for carcinoma than do duct extension and branch pattern.

ovoid and homogeneous, some large fibroadenomas are lobulated and heterogeneous. These large fibroadenomas usually have only two or three gentle lobules (46) (Figs. 11 to 15). The majority of gently lobulated, heterogeneous nodules are larger fibroadenomas. Slightly fewer than 10% of such lesions are ductal carcinomas (usually of the "knobby" type). These frequently have more numerous and smaller microlobules, representing tumor within individual ductal components of the tumor (46,47) (Fig. 16).

Duct extension and *branch pattern* refer to the shape of the nodule. Duct extension represents a projection of the nodule toward the nipple. Branch pattern represents multiple projections from the nodule peripherally away from the nipple. Demonstration of both duct extension and branch pattern requires the primary scan plane to be radially oriented about the nipple and the orthogonal plane to be antiradially oriented (48,49). Some lesions that seem to have only benign characteristics when scanned in the usual longitudinal and transverse planes demonstrate atypical characteristics of duct extension and/or branch pattern when scanned radially and antiradially (Figs. 17 and 18). For this reason all solid nodules should be scanned in radial and antiradial planes. Additionally, using these scan planes in patients whose solid nodules have clear-cut malignant characteristics may help distinguish infiltrating from intraductal components of the cancer, may give a better picture of the true size of the lesion, and may

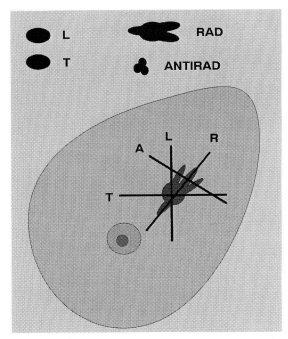

FIG. 18. The importance of radial and antiradial scan planes for the evaluation of solid nodules. The usual longitudinal **(L)** and transverse **(T)** scan planes may show only an ovoid, smooth or a lobulated, heterogeneous nodule with a relatively low chance of malignancy. Radial and antiradial scan planes may show duct extension and/or branch pattern, which have a much greater chance of being associated with malignancy.

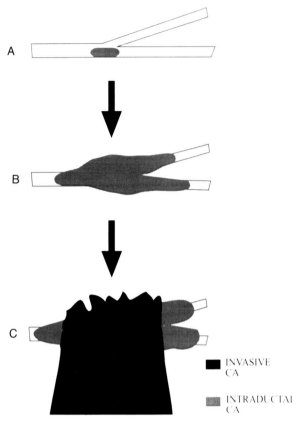

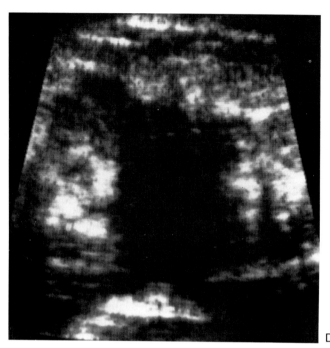

FIG. 19. Schematic representation and ultrasound of mixed infiltrating and intraductal carcinoma. **A:** Small intraductal papillary carcinoma within a normal size duct. **B:** A later stage showing DCIS filling and expanding the duct and extending centripetally toward the nipple and centrifugally away from the nipple but not yet invading. **C:** A later stage in which the the tumor has become invasive at its site of origin but remains intraductal in its duct extensions toward and away from the nipple. **D:** Radial scan showing a central mass of infiltrating ductal carcinoma with duct extensions of noninvasive intraductal tumor toward the nipple (*left*) and away from the nipple (*right*). This corresponds to Stage C in the above schematic. The invasive central mass shows typical malignant features such as angular margins, marked hypoechogenicity, and acoustic shadowing, whereas the noninvasive peripheral intraductal components have sonographically benign characteristics except for their intraductal shape.

help suggest the possibility of an extensive intraductal component (Fig. 19).

BENIGN CHARACTERISTICS OF SOLID NODULES

Benign characteristics of solid nodules each have less than a 5% risk of association with malignancy (8,18,23–25,30,44). These include

- homogeneous echotexture,
- isoechogenicity,
- a well-circumscribed ovoid shape,
- a thin echogenic rim,
- good sound transmission, and
- thin edge shadows.

A nodule must meet all of these criteria to be considered probably benign. A single atypical or malignant characteristic prevents classification as probably benign (Figs. 11 to 20). These solid, probably benign characteristics occur most typically in small fibroadenomas that are frequently less than 1 cm in largest diameter. Larger fibroadenomas tend to become heterogeneous and lobulated. Most of the cancers that may appear benign sonographically are earlier or less aggressive intraductal carcinomas, ductal carcinomas with only microinvasion, or occasional medullary or colloid carcinomas (15,18,26–33) (Fig. 21). Larger and more advanced breast cancers usually have malignant characteristics.

SONOGRAPHIC MISDIAGNOSIS

The Causes of False Negatives

The causes of sonographically missed cancers are geographic miss (whereby the region with the lesion

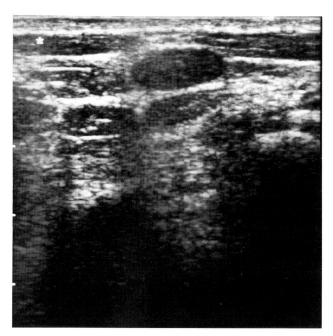

FIG. 20. Fibroadenomas with typically benign features. The typical small fibroadenoma is ovoid, homogeneous, and well circumscribed, with a thin echogenic rim or capsule, good sound transmission, and thin edge shadows.

simply was not scanned), mistaking of the tumor for a fat lobule, inadequate penetration of more superficial dense fibrous tissues, and anechoic appearance due to gain settings that are too low. Most of these mistakes are avoidable with good equipment and sonographic

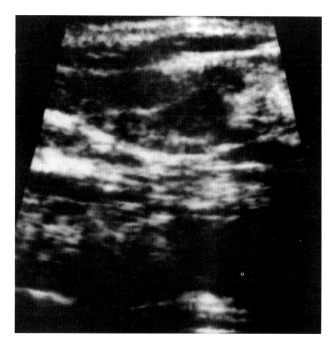

FIG. 21. Ductal carcinoma *in situ* has solid, typically benign sonographic characteristics.

technique and with careful correlation with mammography. Understanding the correlation between sonographic and mammographic findings is the cornerstone of quality breast sonography.

The chances of a geographic miss increase with the extent of the area being scanned. Geographic misses are more likely when the sonogram is not targeted to a specific area of the breast by clinical or mammographic findings. This is one of the reasons that using sonography for screening purposes has not been successful (1,14,15,26,50–53). Compression can improve the image and help in evaluation of the ''hardness'' of lesions. Using such compressive pressure continuously while scanning the breast, however, increases the chances of continually displacing from the beam a mobile lesion of interest and causing a geographic miss.

Most cancers, whether surrounded by fibrous tissue or by fat, are markedly hypoechoic and quite conspicuous. The minority of cancers that are isoechoic, however, may be very difficult to distinguish from surrounding isoechoic fat lobules with sonography alone (5,8,26,28,38,54). It is important to set time-gain curves and overall gain so that fat lobules are a medium-level gray at all depths from the skin to the pectoralis muscles. Inappropriately low gain settings result in darker gray or black fat lobules and make it easier to miss fat-surrounded nodules (38). Additionally, these isoechoic, fat-surrounded lesions are virtually always visible mammographically. It is critical to correlate sonographic and mammographic findings to help avoid missing these lesions. Any *clear-cut* nodule or mass on mammography that cannot be seen with good quality sonographic equipment and technique must be assumed to be solid. It is virtually impossible for careful sonography to miss a cyst that is visible mammographically.

Missing a nodule deep to dense fibrous tissues because of inadequate penetration is rare today, even with 7.5 MHz probes. It was more common with 10 MHz sector water-path probes. Occasionally, however, critical angle shadowing due to obliquely oriented suspensory ligaments or fibrous septa may result in severe shadowing (5,55,56). Usually, this shadowing is pronounced only in one plane and is absent or linear in the orthogonal direction. In such cases the use of an oblique scan plane that is perpendicular to the ligament or septum can diminish shadowing. Heavy compression can also push the shadowing ligament into a plane more perpendicular to the beam and can decrease the thickness of tissue that the beam must penetrate (5). It is especially important to adequately penetrate these areas sonographically because they usually correspond to areas of very dense tissue on mammograms. Lesions are more likely to be missed by mammography in these dense areas than in fatty areas of the breast (53,57,58).

False anechogenicity due to insufficient gain can ar-

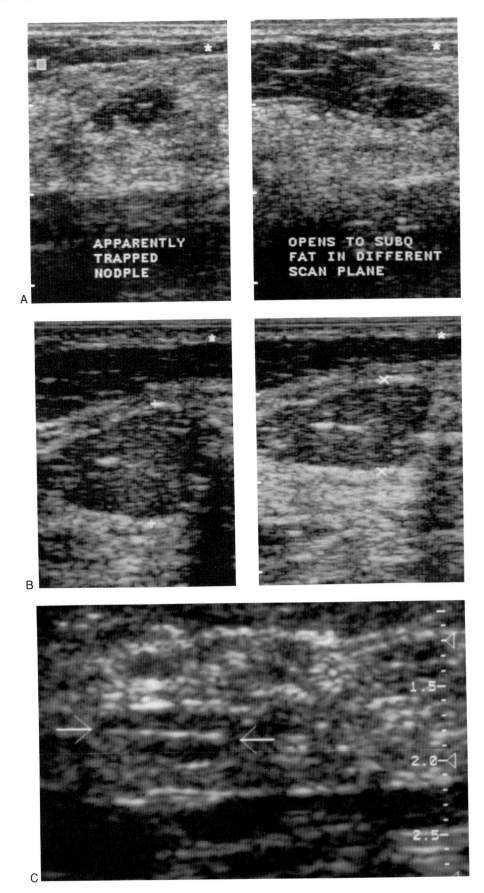

APPARENTLY
TRAPPED
NODPLE

OPENS TO SUBQ
FAT IN DIFFERENT
SCAN PLANE

tificially make solid lesions appear cystic. Two pieces of information will usually be present to help avoid this mistake, however; there will always be a lack of enhanced through-transmission when gain settings have been insufficient, and fat lobules will be too black or dark gray.

The Causes of Sonographic False Positives

Causes of false-positive sonograms are fat lobules, areas of persistent critical angle shadowing, reactive intramammary lymph nodes, cysts too near the skin, filling in of deep cysts due to more superficially located beam-scattering tissues, and excessive gain settings "filling in" cysts. Some people also consider fibroadenomas to be false positives (59). The discovery of fibroadenomas is no different than with mammography, however, and the detection of fibroadenomas by either method should be considered part of the price of improving cancer detection rates. That price—emotional, physical, and economic—is far less for core needle biopsies than it is for excisional biopsies.

Fat lobules, which were mentioned as a cause of false-negative sonography, are also one of the most prominent causes of false-positive sonography (5,8,38). Most fat lobules are contiguous with other adjacent fat lobules, and the connection between them can be demonstrated sonographically in some plane (Fig. 22A). Fat lobules that are completely surrounded by echogenic fibrous tissues may, however, be very difficult to distinguish from pathologic solid nodules. Mammography frequently cannot help us in these cases. These "entrapped" fatty lobules may be obscured by the surrounding water density fibroglandular elements because of the summation effects of mammography. Palpating while scanning and using compression while scanning may be helpful because fat lobules may be soft and deformable (Fig. 22B). Cancers are hard and noncompressible. Fat lobules frequently have a straight, thin echogenic line through their center, the exact origin of which is uncertain (5) (Fig. 22C). This line must be specifically sought by scanning the lobule in multiple planes, since it is visible only in a single random plane. A straight echogenic line such as this is not typically seen in fibroadenomas or cancers. Occasionally, despite all efforts, it is impossible to distinguish a fat lobule from a pathologic solid nodule. Biopsy of these fat lobules is a result of false-positive sonography.

Areas of persistent shadowing due to normal tissues may be difficult to distinguish from malignant shadowing (26,60). The techniques of oblique scan planes and compression discussed above under "The Causes of False Negatives" can also help avoid false-positive scans. Careful correlation with mammographic findings is also essential. Radial scars, large biopsy scars, sclerosing adenosis, and fat necrosis can, however, occasionally cause intense shadowing that cannot be distinguished from malignant shadowing despite all efforts (26,52,60). In such cases, sonography may lead to false-positive diagnoses of cancer.

Intramammary lymph nodes are solid nodules. If they lie in the typical location in the upper outer quadrant and have lucent rims and echogenic hila, a virtually certain diagnosis of intramammary lymph node can be made (61) (a diagnosis as certain as the mammographic demonstration of fat within the hilum) (Fig. 23). Some reactive lymph nodes may be edematous and may not show echogenic hila, however (Fig. 24). If the location and sonographic appearance are not classic, biopsy may be necessary.

Small cysts within the superficial centimeter of the breast may be too near for the elevation plane and transmit zone focusing of the probe (especially with equipment not properly configured for breast ultrasound). Such cysts may also be close enough to the transducer to be influenced by side lobe artifacts. The net effect of this superficial location is "filling in" of the cyst with echoes, making it appear solid (5,8,62–64). Acoustic stand-offs will usually solve this problem (Fig. 18 in Chapter 10). If these artifactual echoes cannot be cleared from the cyst by using a stand-off, however, aspiration or biopsy may be necessary.

Excessive gain settings may cause artifactual echoes within a simple cyst (5,53,60). Clues on the image that may aid in recognizing this technical error are greater enhancement of through-transmission than would be expected with a solid nodule and surrounding fat lobules that appear too echogenic. Similarly, cysts that are deep to beam defocusing tissues may be filled in with scattered sound and may falsely appear solid. Sometimes compression or using a lower frequency transducer can be helpful in clearing these artifactual echoes from the cyst (5).

FIG. 22. Mammary fat lobules. **A:** Split screen image shows a mammary fat lobule that in one plane appears completely entrapped within fibroglandular tissue but in another plane communicates with subcutaneous fat. **B:** Split screen image shows a mammary fat lobule to be soft and partially compressible. Although some fibroadenomas may be partially compressible, cancers are typically very incompressible. **C:** A straight line is demonstrable through the center of a completely entrapped fat lobule. Such straight lines are not seen within fibroadenomas or cancers.

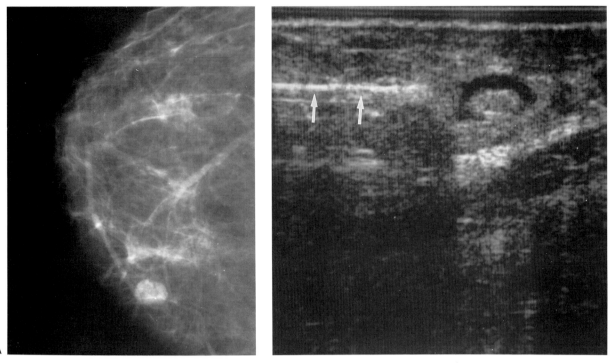

A   B

FIG. 23. Intramammary lymph nodes. **A:** Mammogram shows central fatty density within the hilum of an intramammary lymph node. **B:** Corresponding sonogram shows a sonolucent cortex around the echogenic hilum, which corresponds to the fat density on mammography. This is the typical reniform, "miniature kidney" sonographic appearance of intramammary lymph nodes. The core-biopsy needle is also visible (*arrows*).

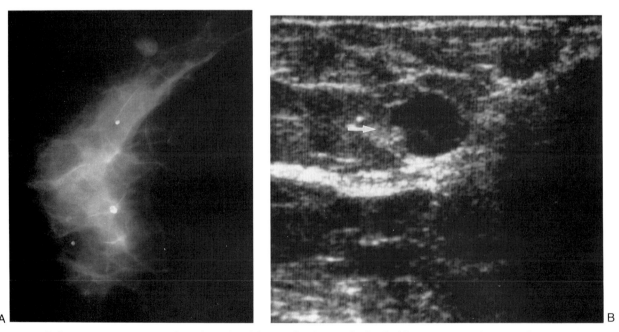

A   B

FIG. 24. Intramammary lymph node with reactive hyperplasia. **A:** Mammogram shows a discrete, well-circumscribed nodule but does not show the central fat typically seen in normal intramammary lymph nodes. The swelling of the node has effaced and obliterated the fat within the hilum. **B:** Sonogram shows findings similar to those of the mammogram. The typical echogenic hilum (*arrow*) is displaced and almost completely obliterated by the swollen cortex. Because the hilum is not demonstrable with certainty, a definitive diagnosis of intramammary lymph node is not possible by mammography or sonography alone. Frequently, the swelling will resolve in a few days to weeks, so short-term follow-up can be done before biopsy.

COLOR DUPLEX SONOGRAPHY OF SOLID BREAST NODULES

Many authors have advocated using Doppler ultrasound to distinguish benign from malignant solid nodules because many breast cancers stimulate the growth of tumor vessels (65–72). Very high frequency continuous wave Doppler probes, duplex sonography, and color duplex sonography have all been used. Cancers have been reported to have higher peak systolic velocities or frequencies and/or lower resistance flow than have benign lesions (65–72). Cancers have been reported to have more vessels within them on color Doppler examination than have benign lesions (73).

Even authors of encouraging studies of the Doppler detection of breast cancer point out that only positive results are helpful (73). Unfortunately, the accuracy of Doppler ultrasound in distinguishing benign from malignant lesions has been disappointing in others' hands (74,75). In fact, color duplex sonography may be less accurate than the two-dimensional (2D) image alone at distinguishing benign from malignant lesions. With highly sensitive color duplex equipment, relatively high velocity, low-resistance flow is found in virtually all solid nodules and occasionally even within normal breast tissue (Fig. 25). We believe that Doppler and color duplex studies of breast nodules should be considered investigational and are not clinically indicated,

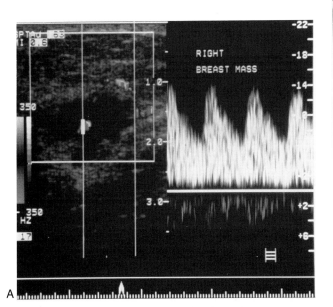

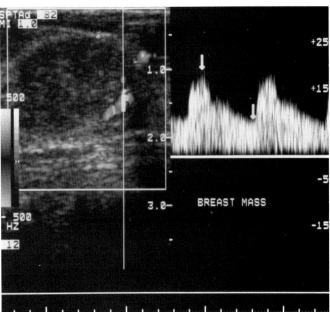

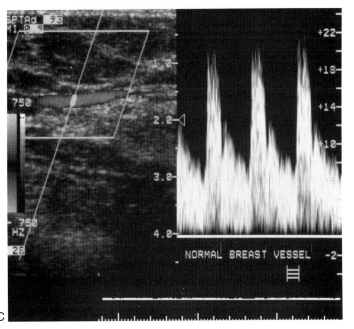

FIG. 25. Color duplex sonography of breast lesions. **A:** Patient 1: Color duplex sonography of breast cancer shows low-resistance flow with peak systolic velocities of 14 cm/sec. **B:** Patient 2: Color duplex sonography of fibroadenoma shows low-resistance flow similar to that of the cancer in A and shows a peak systolic velocity of 19 cm/sec, even higher than that of the cancer. Juvenile fibroadenomas, in particular, may show relatively high-velocity, low-resistance flow. **C:** Patient 3: Flow within a normal breast vessel in a 38-year-old woman on Day 5 of the menstrual cycle.

especially in view of the accuracy, cost effectiveness, and safety of ultrasound-guided core needle biopsies.

CONCLUSION

Breast ultrasound is not a replacement for screening mammography but is a diagnostic tool that supplements mammography in appropriate settings. Although diagnostic mammography is certainly more useful in cases with calcifications and in determining whether a density is real or artifactual, sonographic findings are more definitive than those of diagnostic mammography in most patients with discrete palpable or mammographic nodules and nonspecific focally asymmetric mammographic masses (seen on both MLO and CC views). Breast ultrasound can identify and classify cysts so that further action can be determined. Solid lesions likewise can be evaluated and segregated according to the likelihood of malignancy. If appropriate equipment is used by properly trained personnel, the false negatives and false positives associated with breast sonography can be minimized while overall breast evaluation is dramatically improved.

REFERENCES

1. Sickles EA, Filly RA, Callen PW. Breast cancer detection with sonomammography and mammography: comparison using state-of-the-art equipment. *AJR Am J Roentgenol* 1983;140:843–845.
2. Jellins J, Kossoff G, Reeve TS, Barraclough BH. Detection and classification of liquid-filled masses in the breast by gray-scale echography. *Radiology* 1975;125:205–212.
3. Hilton SW, Leopold GR, Olson LK, et al. Real-time breast sonography: application in 300 consecutive patients. *AJR Am J Roentgenol* 1986;147:479–486.
4. Sickles EA, Filly RA, Callen PW. Benign breast lesions: ultrasound detection and diagnosis. *Radiology* 1984;151:467–470.
5. Bassett LW, Kimme-Smith C. Breast sonography: technique, equipment, and normal anatomy. *Semin Ultrasound CT MR* 1989;10(2):82–89.
6. Basset LW, Kimme-Smith C. Breast sonography. *AJR Am J Roentgenol* 1991;156:449–455.
7. Feig SA. The role of ultrasound in a breast imaging center. *Semin Ultrasound CT MR* 1989;10:90–105.
8. Adler DD. Ultrasound of benign breast conditions. *Semin Ultrasound CT MR* 10:106–118.
9. Tabar L, Pentek Z, Dean PB. The diagnostic and therapeutic value of breast cyst puncture and pneumocystography. *Radiology* 1981;141:659.
10. Reuter K, D'Orsi CJ, Reale F. Intracystic carcinoma of the breast: the role of ultrasonography. *Radiology* 1984;153:233–234.
11. Estabrook A, Asch T, Gump F, et al. Mammographic features of intracystic papillary lesions. *Surg Gynecol Obstet* 1990;170:113–116.
12. Barki Y, Benharroch D, Vinograd L, Hoda G. Infarcted cystadenofibroma of the breast: ultrasonic appearance. *J Ultrasound Med* 1987;6:213–215.
13. Hayashi N, Tamaki N, Honekura Y, et al. Real-time sonography of palpable breast masses. *Br J Radiol* 1985;58:611–615.
14. Kopans DB, Meyer JE, Lindfors KK. Whole-breast ultrasound imaging: four year follow-up. *Radiology* 1985;157:505–507.
15. Bassett LW, Kimme-Smith C, Sutherland LK, et al. Automated
16. and hand-held breast ultrasound: effect on patient management. *Radiology* 1987;165:103–108.
16. Dempsey PJ. The importance of resolution in the clinical application of the breast sonography. *Ultrasound Med Biol* 1988;14(1):43–48.
17. Croll J, Kotevich J, Tabretet M. The diagnosis of benign disease and the exclusion of malignancy in patients with breast symptoms. *Semin Ultrasound CT MR* [in press].
18. Cole-Beuglet C, Soriano RZ, Kurtz AB, Goldberg BB. Ultrasound analysis of 104 primary breast carcinomas classified according to histopathologic type. *Radiology* 1983;147:191–196.
19. Jellins J, Reeve TS, Croll J, Kossoff G. Results of breast echographic examinations in Sydney, Australia, 1972–1979. *Semin Ultrasound CT MR* 1982;3:58–62.
20. Egan RL, Egan KL. Detection of breast carcinoma: comparison of automated water-path whole-breast sonography, mammography, and physical examination. *AJR Am J Roentgenol* 1984;143:493–497.
21. Smallwood JA, Guyer P, Dewbury K, et al. The accuracy of ultrasound in the diagnosis of breast disease. *Ann R Coll Surg Engl* 1986;68:19–22.
22. Van Dam PA, Van Goethem MLA, Kersschot E, et al. Palpable solid breast masses: retrospective single and multimodality evaluation of 201 lesions. *Radiology* 1988;166:435–439.
23. Cole-Beuglet C, Soriano RZ, Durtz AB, et al. Fibroadenoma of the breast: sonomammography correlated in 122 patients. *AJR Am J Roentgenol* 1983;140:369–375.
24. Jackson VP, Rothschild PA, Krepke DL, et al. The spectrum of sonographic findings of fibroadenoma of the breast. *Invest Radiol* 1986;21:34–40.
25. Heywang SH, Lipsit ER, Glassman LM, et al. Specificity of ultrasonography in the diagnosis of benign breast masses. *J Ultrasound Med* 1984;3:453–461.
26. Jackson VP. Sonography of malignant breast disease. *Semin Ultrasound CT MR* 1989;10(2):119–131.
27. Kobayashi T. Diagnostic ultrasound in breast cancer: analysis of retrotumorous echo patterns correlated with sonic attenuation by cancerous connective tissue. *J Clin Ultrasound* 1979;7:471–479.
28. Maturo VG, Zusmer NR, Gilson AJ, Bear B. Ultrasonic appearance of mammary carcinoma with a dedicated whole-breast scanner [in press].
29. Jellins J, Reeve TS, Kossoff G. *Clin Diagn Ultrasound* 1984;12:25–39.
30. Harper AP, Kelly-Fry E, Noe JS, Bies JR, Jackson VP. Ultrasound in the evaluation of solid breast masses. *Radiology* 1983;146:731–736.
31. McSweeney MB, Murphy CH. Whole-breast sonography. *Radiol Clin North Am* 1985;23:157–167.
32. Kasumi F, Fukami A, Kuno K, et al. Characteristic echographic features of circumscribed cancer. *Ultrasound Med Biol* 1982;8:369–375.
33. Meyer JE, Amin E, Lindfors KK, et al. Medullary carcinoma of the breast: mammographic and ultrasound appearance. *Radiology* 1989;170:79.
34. Baum G. Ultrasound mammography. *Radiology* 1977;122:199–205.
35. Cole-Beuglet C, Goldberg BB, Kurtz AB, et al. Clinical experience with a prototype real-time dedicated breast scanner. *AJR Am J Roentgenol* 1982;139:905–911.
36. Field S, Dunn F. Correlation of echographic visibility of tissue with biological composition and physiological state. *J Acoust Soc Am* 1973;54:809.
37. Calderon C, Vikomerson D, Mezrich R, et al. Differences in the attenuation of ultrasound by normal, benign, and malignant breast tissue. *J Clin Ultrasound* 1976;4:249–254.
38. Jackson VP, Kelly-Fry E, Rothschild PA, et al. Automated breast sonography using a 7.5 mHz PVDF transducer: preliminary clinical evaluation. *Radiology* 1986;159:679–684.
39. Sickles EA. Sonographic detection of breast calcifications. In: Fullerton GD, ed. *Applications of optical instrumentation in medicine: XI. Proceedings of SPIE, the International Society for Optical Engineering.* Bellingham, WA: International Society for Optical Engineering; 1983;419:51–52.

40. Lambie RW, Hodgden D, Herman EM. Sonomammographic manifestations of mammographically detectable breast microcalcifications. *J Ultrasound Med* 1983;2:509–514.

41. Kopans DB, Meyer JE, Steinbbock RT. Breast cancer: the appearance as delineated by whole breast water-path ultrasound scanning. *J Clin Ultrasound* 1982;10:313–322.

42. Kasumi F, Tanaka H. Detection of microcalcifications in breast carcinoma by ultrasound. In: Jellins J, Kobayashi T, eds. *Ultrasonic examination of the breast.* New York: Wiley; 1983:89–97.

43. Adler DD, Hyde DL, Ikeda DM. Quantitative sonographic parameters as a means of distinguishing breast cancers from benign solid breast masses. *J Ultrasound Med* 1991;10:505–508.

44. Fornage BD, Lorigan JG, Andry E. Fibroadenoma of the breast: sonographic appearance. *Radiology* 1989;172:671.

45. Nishimura S, Matsusue S, Koezumi S, et al. Size of breast cancer on ultrasonography, cut-surface of resected specimen, and palpation. *Ultrasound Med Biol* 1988;14:139.

46. Sickles EA. Breast masses: mammographic evaluation. *Radiology* 1989;173:297–303.

47. Martin JE. *Atlas of mammography.* 1st ed. Baltimore: Williams & Wilkins; 1982.

48. Rosenweig R, Foy PM, Cole-Beuglet C, et al. Radial scanning of the breast: an alternative to the standard ultrasound technique. *J Clin Ultrasound* 1982;10:199–201.

49. Baum G. Labeling of meridional and radial scans of the breast. *J Ultrasound Med* 1982;1:105–110.

50. Moskowitz M. Screening is not diagnosis. *Radiology* 1979;133:265–268.

51. ACR Committee on Breast Imaging. *Policy statement on sonography for the detection and diagnosis of breast disease,* Reston, VA, 1984.

52. Dempsey PJ, Moskowitz M. Is there a role for breast sonography? *Clin Diagn Ultrasound* 1987;20:17–36.

53. Jackson VP. The role of ultrasound in breast imaging. *Radiology* 1990;177:305–311.

54. Kimme-Smith C, Bassett LW, Gold RH. High frequency breast ultrasound: hand-held versus screening. *J Ultrasound Med* 1988;7:77–81.

55. Schenck CD, Lehman DA. Sonographic anatomy of the breast. *Semin Ultrasound* 1982;3:13–33.

56. Kossoff G, Jellins J. The physics of breast echography. *Semin Ultrasound* 1982;3:5–12.

57. Kalisher L. Factors influencing false negative rates in xeromammography. *Radiology* 1979;133:297–301.

58. Martin J, Moskowitz M, Milbrath JR. Breast cancers missed by mammography. *AJR Am J Roentgenol* 1979;132:737–739.

59. Kopans DB. What is a useful adjunct to mammography? *Radiology* 1986;161:560–561.

60. Hayashi N, Tamaki N, Honekura Y, et al. Real-time sonography of palpable breast masses. *Br J Radiol* 1985;58:611–615.

61. Gordon PB, Gilkes B. Sonographic appearance of normal intramammary lymph nodes. *J Ultrasound Med* 1988;7:545–548.

62. Rubin E, Miller VE, Berland LL, et al. Hand-held real-time breast sonography. *AJR Am J Roentgenol* 1985;14:623–629.

63. Kimme-Smith C, Hansen M, Bassett LW, et al. Ultrasound mammography effects of focal zone placement. *Radiographics* 1985;5:955–970.

64. Kimme-Smith C, Rothschild PA, Bassett LW, et al. Ultrasound artifacts affect the diagnosis of breast masses. *Ultrasound Med Biol* 1988;14[Suppl 1]:103–210.

65. Wells PNT, Halliwell M, Skidmore R, et al. Tumour detection by ultrasonic Doppler blood-flow signals. *Ultrasonics* 1977;15:231–232.

66. White DN, Cledgett PR. Breast carcinoma detection by ultrasonic Doppler signals. *Ultrasound Med Biol* 1978;4:329–335.

67. Burns PN, Halliwell M, Wells PNT, Webb AJ. Ultrasonic Doppler studies of the breast. *Ultrasound Med Biol* 1982;8:127–143.

68. Minasian H, Bamber JC. A preliminary assessment of an ultrasonic Doppler method for the study of blood flow in human breast cancer. *Ultrasound Med Biol* 1982;8:357–364.

69. Halliwell M, Burns PN, Wells PNT. An ultrasonic duplex breast scanner. *Ultrasound Med Biol* 1982;8(1):72.

70. Jellins J, Kossoff G, Gill RW, Reeve TS. Combined B-mode and Doppler examination of the breast. *Ultrasound Med Biol* 1982;8(1):89.

71. Schoenberger SG, Sutherland CM, Robinson AE. Breast neoplasms: duplex sonographic imaging as an adjunct in diagnosis. *Radiology* 1988;168:665–668.

72. Dock W. Duplex sonography of mammary tumors: a prospective study of 75 patients. *J Ultrasound Med* [in press].

73. Cosgrove DO, Bamber JC, Davey JB, et al. Color Doppler signals from breast tumors: work in progress. *Radiology* 1990;176:175–180.

74. Jackson VP. Duplex sonography of the breast. *Ultrasound Med Biol* 1988;14:(1):131–137.

75. Barraclough BM, Picker RH, Barraclough BH. Whole breast ultrasound mammography: a useful modality in screening for breast cancer. In: Jellins J, Kossoff G, Croll J, eds. *Proceedings of the Fourth International Congress on the Ultrasonic Examination of the Breast.* St. Leonards, Australia; 1985:159–166.

Percutaneous Breast Biopsy, edited by
Steve H. Parker and William E. Jobe.
Raven Press, Ltd., New York © 1993.

CHAPTER 12

Interventional Breast Ultrasound

Steve H. Parker and A. Thomas Stavros

Until recently, virtually all breast interventions were performed by surgeons. The participation of radiologists was limited to the interpretation of mammograms, often of dubious quality. In the past few years, mammography and ultrasound have improved significantly, and specialized needles for injection, localization, aspiration, and biopsy have been developed. These technological advances have created the potential for drastic changes in the radiologist's role in breast intervention. As its full potential is realized, ultrasound will be at the forefront of the changes.

Previously, ultrasound was used in the breast primarily to distinguish between cystic and solid lesions. Despite vast improvements in the technology, breast ultrasound has not gained wide acceptance yet and is still infrequently used in diagnostic applications.

Recently, high-frequency, electronically focused, linear and convex array ultrasound transducers were developed to improve near-field imaging. As a result, breast ultrasound can now be used for much more than mere cyst vs. solid differentiation. With modern ultrasound, palpable breast lesions can be characterized as simple or complex cysts, fibrosis, areas of fibrocystic change, or solid lesions of varying malignant probability (see Chapter 11). Many nonpalpable, mammographic lesions can be further characterized with ultrasound. Also, some lesions not suspected on mammography can be identified ultrasonographically (Fig. 1) (see Chapters 10 and 11). Perhaps most importantly, radiologists can use ultrasound to guide breast cyst aspiration, abscess drainage, needle localization, and percutaneous needle biopsy.

Unfortunately, the longstanding division between interventional radiologists, ultrasonologists, and mam-

mographers has limited the cooperation between their subspecialties. Interventionalists, traditionally poorly trained in ultrasound, tend to use fluoroscopy and CT almost exclusively for guiding procedures and know little about breast disease. Radiologists who specialize in ultrasound tend not to perform interventional procedures and likewise are not typically interested in the breast. Perhaps the most unfortunate situation exists in the breast imaging field itself, where mammographers have typically shied far away from ultrasound and interventional radiology. This situation probably will change as more interventional fellowships and residency programs in radiology emphasize the use of ultrasound in breast disease.

Normal breast ultrasound, abnormal breast ultrasound, and ultrasound-guided core biopsy are covered in Chapters 10, 11, and 13, respectively.

EQUIPMENT

The needles used for aspiration, drainage, and localization are different for each interventional procedure. The ultrasound equipment necessary for each of these is the same, however.

As with diagnostic applications, the ultrasound equipment used in breast intervention is critical to the success of the procedure. Many manufacturers make ultrasound equipment that can be used in the breast. It has been erroneously stated, however, that any low-cost ultrasound equipment is adequate (1). As noted earlier, the equipment must be state of the art with high-frequency, electronically focused, linear array transducers capable of producing excellent near-field images (see Chapter 10). It is extremely helpful if the transducer is compact and lightweight (Fig. 2). Heavy, large, bulky transducers are not suitable for ultrasound-guided breast intervention. Price alone does not ensure high-quality near-field imaging, since machines

S.H. Parker and A.T. Stavros: Radiology Imaging Associates, Breast Diagnostic and Counseling Centre, Englewood, Colorado 80111.

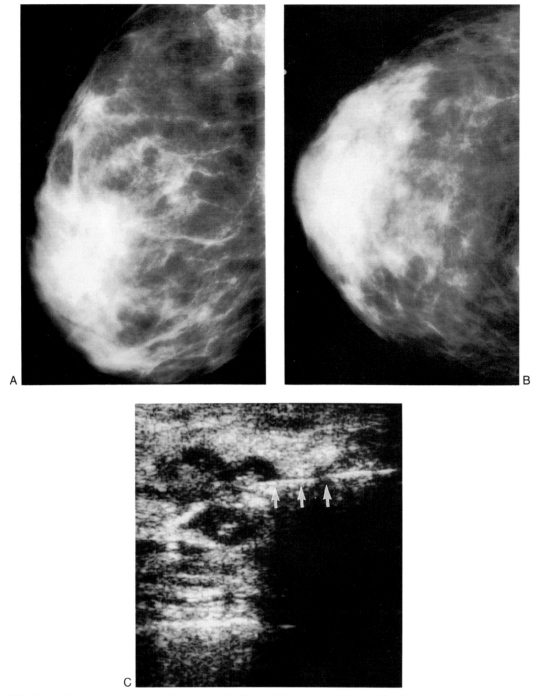

FIG. 1. Lesion seen only on ultrasound. **A:** Mediolateral view demonstrating only dense subareolar and periareolar tissue. **B:** Craniocaudal view likewise demonstrates no evidence of a discrete lesion. **C:** Ultrasound revealed a heart-shaped, solid lesion. Therefore, ultrasound-guided core biopsy was performed. The core needle (*arrows*) is in the prefire position. The histologic diagnosis was infiltrating ductal carcinoma. (From Parker et al., Ref. *1a,* with permission.)

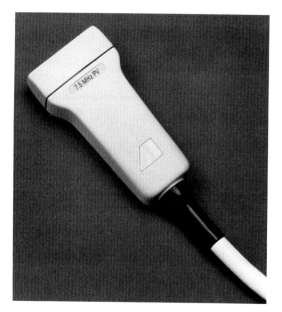

FIG. 2. Small, compact, lightweight linear array transducer from Acoustic Imaging (AI) (Acoustic Imaging, Phoenix, Arizona). The transducer can be soaked in disinfectant solution in its entirety right up to the cord.

costing over $200,000 are still not adequate for good breast ultrasound (Fig. 3). Equipment must be evaluated on an image basis rather than on a price basis.

Frequently, old, outdated ultrasound equipment is retired from the general ultrasound section to the breast section, probably because of a lack of ultrasound experience on the part of the radiologists responsible for breast imaging. Using suboptimal equipment in the breast where image quality is critical creates a never-ending cycle. Inexperienced radiologists who do not have access to the kind of equipment that would allow them to improve their skills are unable to recognize that better equipment is necessary. When economy is a consideration, older ultrasound equipment that provides adequate images of deeper, larger organs such as gallbladder and uterus can continue to be used in that capacity. However, these machines do not provide the high-resolution, near-field images needed to evaluate the comparatively smaller, more superficial lesions in the breast. Good breast ultrasound is virtually impossible without state-of-the-art equipment.

TECHNIQUE

Ultrasound-guided interventions in the breast can be performed in the same way as ultrasound-guided interventions in other anatomic sites. Three methods are

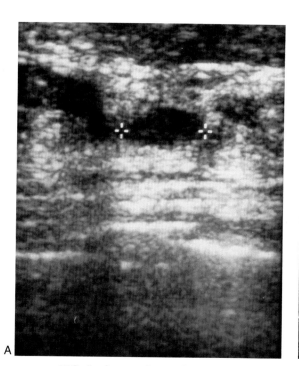

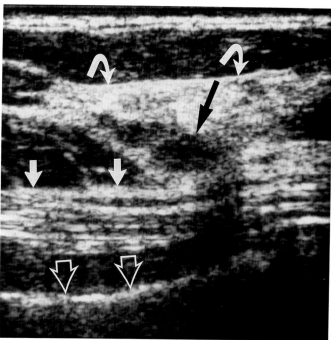

FIG. 3. Comparison of ultrasound images of the same lesion with two different pieces of ultrasound equipment. **A:** "Solid" lesion (*electronic cursors*) found with a nationally known ultrasound unit and referred to the BDCC for biopsy. **B:** Same area scanned with an AI 5200 revealed that the lesion was merely a part of a fat lobule (*long arrow*). Therefore, no biopsy was performed. In addition, the tissue planes (*curved arrows*), the pectoralis muscle (*short arrows*), and the pleural surface of the lung (*open arrows*) are better delineated on the AI image.

available: the memory, biopsy guide, and freehand techniques. The method chosen depends on each radiologist's individual experience and training.

The memory technique involves locating the lesion, measuring the depth from the skin with ultrasound, and then marking the overlying skin with indelible ink. The needle is advanced to the determined depth through the point marked on the skin. Not visualizing the needle as it traverses the lesion is the disadvantage of the memory technique. If the needle deflects off a fibrous region in its path or if the lesion itself moves away from the needle, the operator may not realize that the needle has strayed from its intended course. Without imaging, there is no way to confirm accurate targeting. Thus, the memory technique is not much more effective than the surgeon's "blind," manual interventions guided by palpation.

Biopsy guides, available for most transducers, can be used for breast interventions as well. With biopsy guides the radiologist can visualize the needle as it traverses the lesion. The guides can be somewhat cumbersome, though, and create sterility concerns. More importantly, however, they limit the angle at which a lesion can be approached. This may prohibit using the best pathway to the lesion while avoiding the chest wall.

The freehand technique, which eliminates the disadvantages of the memory and needle-guide techniques, is the most successful method elsewhere in the body (2) (Fig. 4). With the freehand technique, the radiologist holds the transducer in one hand and the needle in the other. The transducer is positioned so that the lesion is near the center of the image. The needle is placed underneath the long axis of the transducer at a very horizontal angle. The flat angle of approach places the needle nearly parallel to the transducer face and nearly perpendicular to the ultrasound beam. This cre-

ates a strong specular reflector, which dramatically improves needle visualization.

The freehand technique allows continuous observation of the needle and lesion without the constraints of a needle guide. However, this is true only if the needle is placed under the long axis of the transducer. Some investigators have advocated approaching the lesion under the short axis of the transducer, but this is not much better than the memory technique because the needle cannot be seen as it is advanced through the breast. With the proper long-axis, freehand technique, the lesion can be approached at virtually any angle (Fig. 5), even parallel to the chest wall. The freehand technique does, however, require more skill and experience than does the needle-guide technique. Before performing the procedure on patients, radiologists can practice on phantoms to master the freehand approach.

Regardless of the technique used, the radiologist must plan an appropriate route of approach after locating the lesion. Several factors are important, including the depth of the lesion, the angle of the chest wall, and the presence and amount of dense fibrous tissue in the vicinity of the lesion. The depth of the lesion influences the angle of approach. From a technical standpoint, superficial lesions are generally the easiest to target. Superficial lesions can be approached more parallel to the transducer than can deeper lesions, while still maintaining a relatively direct route (Fig. 5A). Deeper lesions require a less parallel, more oblique approach, which makes it more difficult to visualize the needle. Normally, the transducer is positioned with the lesion in the center of the image. With deep lesions, however, the transducer is positioned with the lesion to the side of the image (i.e., the lesion is visualized on one end of the transducer, and the needle entry point is visualized on the other) (Fig. 5B). In this way the course of the needle will be as close to parallel as possible, ensuring the best needle visualization. As the periphery of the lesion is approached, the needle can be levered downward. This compresses the outer portion of the breast and brings the needle more parallel to the transducer, further enhancing needle visualization (Fig. 6A). Thus, deeper lesions require a skin entry point slightly further from the lesion so that the needle can move as close as possible to a horizontal course.

Lesions close to or abutting the chest wall can be targeted with ultrasound guidance but pose some additional problems that require altering the route. With appropriate planning, however, they can be approached confidently and safely.

One way to approach chest wall lesions would be to move the skin entry point well away from the lesion to assume a course more parallel to the chest wall (Fig. 6B). This approach has two drawbacks, however. First, the farther the skin entry point is from the transducer, the harder it is to observe the needle and keep

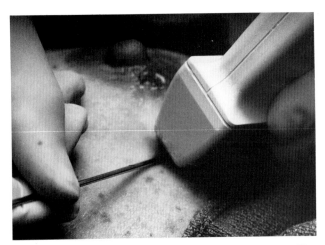

FIG. 4. Freehand technique of ultrasound guidance. The same operator holds the needle in one hand and the transducer in the other.

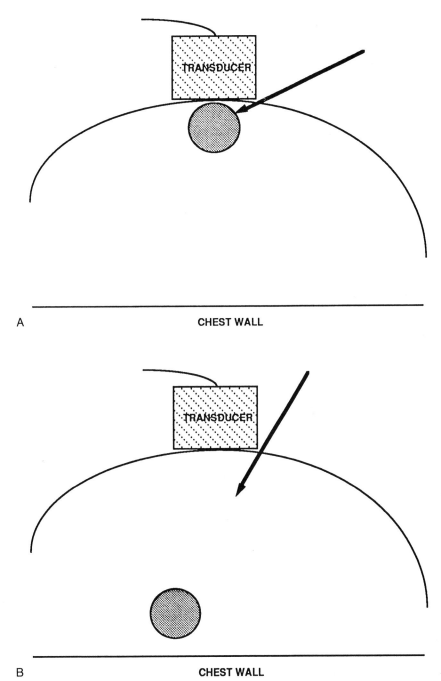

A   CHEST WALL

B   CHEST WALL

FIG. 5. Schematic representation of the different approaches used with freehand guidance. **A:** Superficial lesion approached nearly parallel to the transducer. **B:** Deeper lesion requiring more of an oblique angle.

it in the plane of the ultrasound beam, since direct physical contact with the end of the transducer is lost and the initial path is blind to the transducer. Second, this approach creates a longer needle tract than the more direct oblique approach.

Thus, for most chest wall lesions, the oblique approach used for other deep lesions is preferable. Since the needle enters the skin at a relatively steep angle, as close to the transducer as possible, a medial to lateral (rather than lateral to medial) approach takes advan-

tage of the chest wall's natural curvature. Again, this involves positioning the transducer with the lesion on one side and the skin entry point on the other. Instilling local anesthetic into the region between the lesion and the chest wall can raise the lesion somewhat. Then, by introducing the biopsy needle into the space between the lesion and the chest wall and levering it downward, one can compress the underlying breast tissue along the shaft of the needle. This creates an approach more parallel to the chest wall (Fig. 6A).

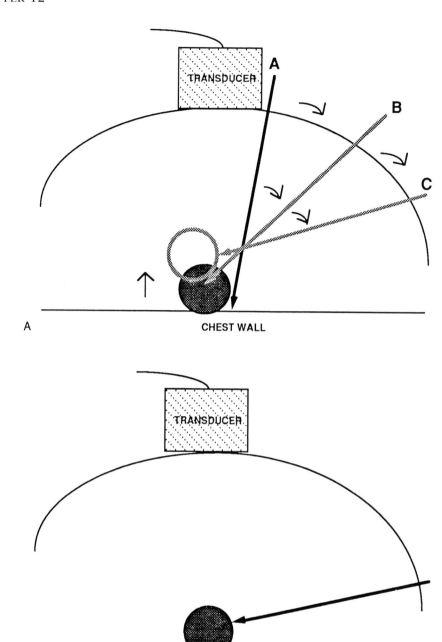

FIG. 6. Schematic representation of possible approaches for deep or chest wall lesions. **A:** With the lever method, the needle approaches the lesion at a relatively steep angle. Then the needle is levered for better visualization and avoidance of the chest wall. **B:** The parallel method requires moving the skin entry point away from the transducer. This makes it more difficult to stay in line with the ultrasound beam and usually requires traversing more tissue. (From Parker et al., Ref. 1a, with permission.)

Finally, a route that minimizes the amount of fibro-glandular tissue traversed is recommended whenever possible for all breast interventions. Fibroglandular tissue is "rubbery," is difficult to penetrate, and may act as a blunt wedge that pushes the lesion out of the way. Also, it typically is more sensitive than fat-replaced regions of the breast.

After the lesion has been located and a route of approach planned, final preparations can be completed. The skin is prepped with povidone-iodine, the transducer is soaked in standard antiseptic cleansing solution, and sterile jelly is applied to the breast. Sterile transducer drapes are not recommended as they severely degrade the resolution of small-parts images. The skin and chosen needle tract are then anesthetized (see Chapter 13).

Local anesthetics are normally acidic and produce a stinging sensation. Mixing sodium bicarbonate with the local anesthetic neutralizes the acidity, preventing the "sting" (see Chapter 4). With any ultrasound-guided intervention, all the patient should feel is the initial skin prick of the small-gauge anesthetic needle. Because the patient feels no discomfort with the injection of local anesthetic, there is no reason to avoid its liberal use in ultrasound-guided interventions. [Unlike the situation with stereotactic mammography, the anesthetic does not obscure ultrasonographic visualization of the lesion (Fig. 9A).]

In fact, no matter what kind of ultrasound-guided intervention is planned, liberal use of local anesthetic is strongly advised. While observing the anesthetic needle, the radiologist becomes familiar with the angle of approach and depth of puncture that will be required for the ensuing intervention. Since the administration of local anesthetic takes only a few moments and can improve patient tolerance and cooperation, it is a small investment to make to ensure a comfortable, successful procedure.

The specifics of ultrasound-guided cyst aspiration, abscess drainage, and needle localization are described below. Ultrasound-guided core biopsy is described in Chapter 13.

CYST ASPIRATION

Although the cause of breast cysts is not entirely clear, they seem to arise in distended lobular units of terminal ducts. As the lobular units unfold and fuse, hypersecretion of fluid creates progressively larger spaces. A single large cyst is formed from the coalescence of former lobules (3).

In some practices, all cysts are aspirated based on the theory that certain biochemical and cytologic characteristics of cysts are markers for increased breast cancer risk (4). This theory has not been proven, however. Therefore, at the Breast Diagnostic and Counseling Centre the main indications for aspiration of simple breast cysts remain patient discomfort or a confusing mammogram.

Complex cysts, on the other hand, are universally viewed with greater suspicion. These cysts should be aspirated and then biopsied if the aspiration is unsuccessful, regardless of patient symptoms or indeterminate mammography (Fig. 7).

Sometimes it is difficult to determine ultrasonographically whether or not a complex cyst is merely a cluster of smaller simple cysts or a necrotic or mucinous neoplasm. Some complex cysts that are composed of numerous simple cysts can be aspirated because the cysts communicate with each other. Others cannot be aspirated because the cysts do not communicate with each other, and each component cyst has too little fluid. Such nonaspirable lesions should be treated as if they were solid.

Aspirations of palpable breast lesions have traditionally been performed by clinicians (usually surgeons) in their offices using a needle with a syringe attached to create vacuum and collect the fluid. As an essentially "blind" procedure, manual aspiration has significant limitations. Palpability does not guarantee that a lump is cystic rather than solid (5) and cannot ensure that the needle definitely enters the lesion. Without the clinician's awareness, the aspiration needle can wander off course and never strike the target, even if it is a simple cyst. There is no way to confirm that the syringe actually contains a representative sample of the lesion or that, if the lesion is a cyst, it has been completely drained. Even when fluid is obtained, without image guidance there is no way to evaluate for complete evacuation, complexity, or possible association with a cancer. Unsuccessful manual cyst aspiration thus subjects the patient to one or more needle sticks without gaining any further information about her lesion.

Ultrasound, on the other hand, provides significantly more information than palpation. Following a needle with continuous ultrasound guidance ensures accurate targeting and complete evacuation during aspiration (5) (Fig. 8).

Once confirmed with ultrasound, cysts are aspirated at the BDCC using the freehand technique described above. Standard 21 gauge Vacutainer phlebotomy needles with red top tubes are preferred for the ensuing aspiration because they eliminate the need to attach a separate syringe (5). As soon as the skin is punctured, the red top tube can be advanced into the needle hub, creating vacuum. The needle is then guided toward the cyst and the cyst is drained automatically. Alternatively, advancing the needle into the cyst before activating the vacuum allows ultrasound documentation of

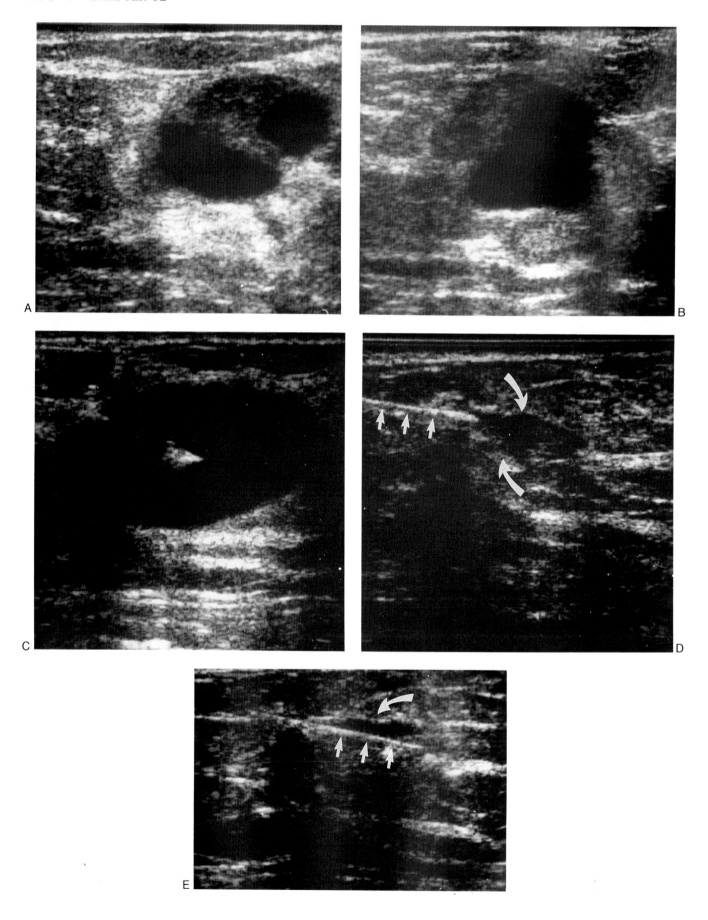

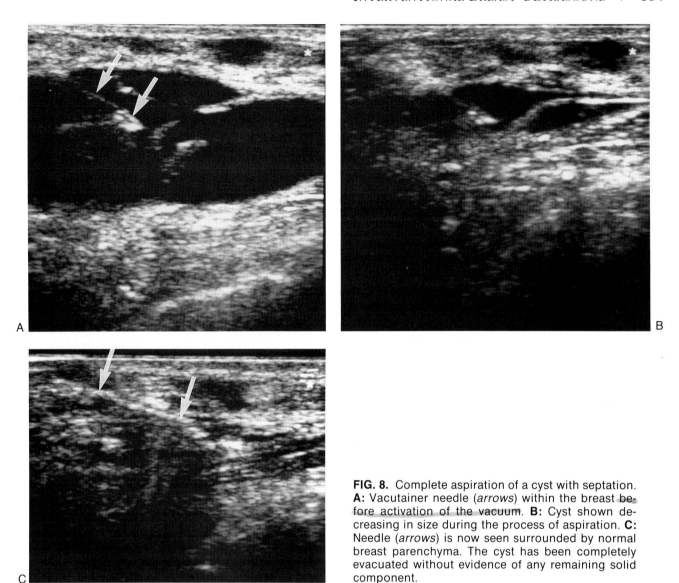

FIG. 8. Complete aspiration of a cyst with septation. **A:** Vacutainer needle (*arrows*) within the breast before activation of the vacuum. **B:** Cyst shown decreasing in size during the process of aspiration. **C:** Needle (*arrows*) is now seen surrounded by normal breast parenchyma. The cyst has been completely evacuated without evidence of any remaining solid component.

FIG. 7. Complex cyst workup in a 28-year-old pregnant patient. **A:** Transverse image of the complex cyst. **B:** Sagittal view. **C:** Vacutainer needle within the cystic portion just before aspiration. **D:** Solid component remaining (*curved arrows*) after aspiration and targeted by a 14 gauge core needle (*short arrows*). **E:** The postfire image shows a needle (*short arrows*) coursing through the remaining solid component (*curved arrow*). The cytology of the cystic component was benign, whereas the core histology of the solid component showed carcinoma. If the patient had been worked up with "blind" (without ultrasound guidance) clinical aspiration, the results would have been disastrously misleading.

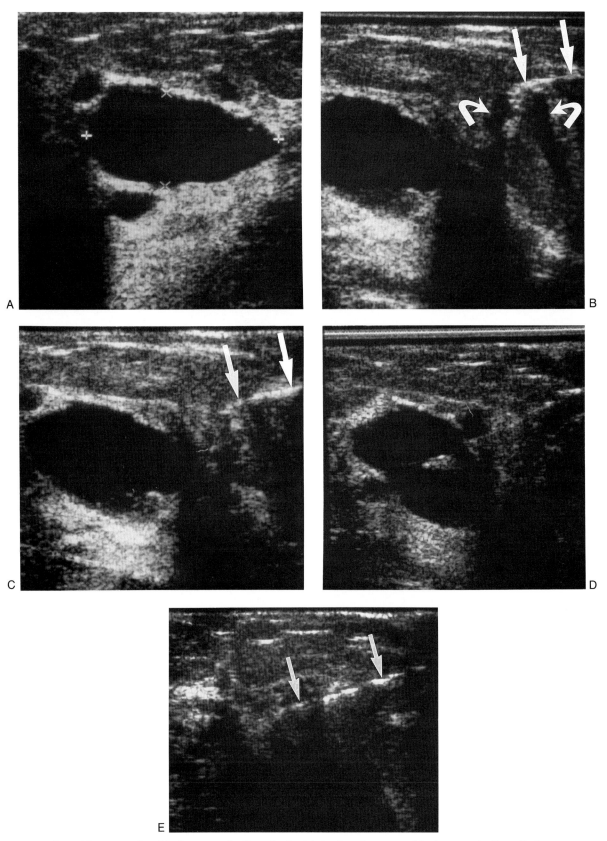

FIG. 9. Ultrasound-guided cyst aspiration. **A:** Cyst (*electronic cursors*) before aspiration. **B:** Anesthetic needle (*long arrows*) depositing anesthetic (*curved arrows*) along the expected path of the Vacutainer needle. **C:** Vacutainer needle (*arrows*) immediately follows the anesthetic needle toward the cyst. **D:** Documentation of the needle within the cyst before activation of the vacuum. **E:** Cyst has been entirely evacuated, and needle (*arrows*) can be withdrawn. (From Parker et al., Ref. *5a*, with permission.)

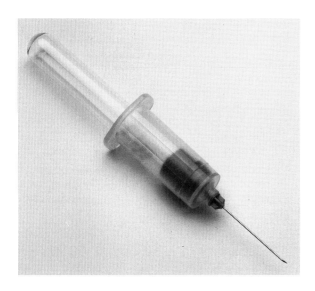

FIG. 10. Standard Vacutainer needle and red top tube. (Courtesy of Geoffrey Wheeler.)

the needle in the cyst before and after aspiration (Fig. 9). Using a Vacutainer needle decreases the length of the cyst aspiration procedure, which in turn decreases patient discomfort (Fig. 10).

For deep cysts in large breasts, the standard Vacutainer needle may not be long enough. Recently introduced adapters allow the attachment of a spinal needle, which should be long enough to reach any cyst within the breast (5) (Fig. 11).

After ultrasound-guided cyst aspiration, it is sometimes fruitful to perform a postaspiration mammogram to prove that the mammographic lesion has resolved (Fig. 12). In patients with multiple bilateral cysts that prevent good mammographic visualization of the breast parenchyma, extensive bilateral cyst aspiration can be followed by mammography. This usually results in a much more interpretable mammogram (Fig. 13).

Some patients may have many indeterminate lesions bilaterally. It is certainly much easier for these patients to undergo sequential ultrasound-guided aspiration and core biopsy than to have each lesion surgically biopsied. Another option is to aspirate and biopsy the largest lesion(s) on each side and then follow the remainder with mammography and ultrasound in six months. Finally, some patients and their physicians may simply desire only short-interval follow-up of multiple lesions.

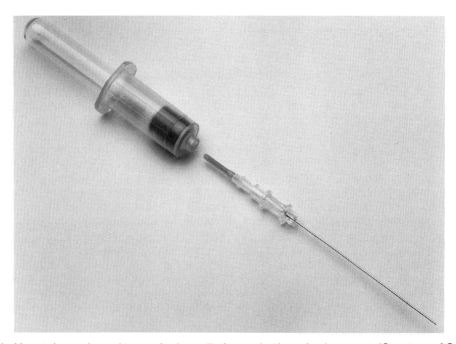

FIG. 11. Vacutainer adapted to a spinal needle for aspiration of a deep cyst. (Courtesy of Geoffrey Wheeler.)

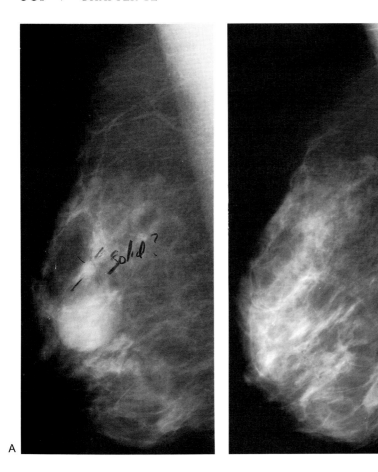

FIG. 12. Resolution of mammographic lesions after cyst aspiration. **A:** Preaspiration mediolateral view demonstrating two densities, one of which was thought to be possibly solid on ultrasound examination. **B:** Postaspiration mediolateral view showing resolution of both mammographic lesions.

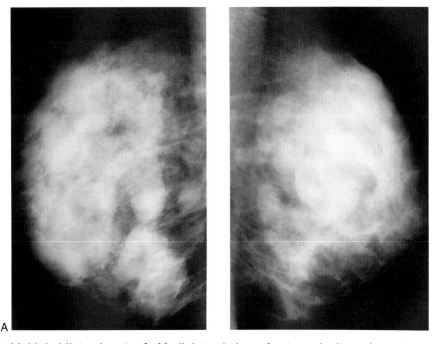

FIG. 13. Multiple bilateral cysts. **A:** Mediolateral view of extremely dense breasts secondary to numerous bilateral densities that were shown to be cysts on ultrasound. **B:** Preaspiration craniocaudal view. **C:** Mediolateral view after ultrasound-guided aspiration of the bilateral cysts. **D:** Postaspiration craniocaudal view.

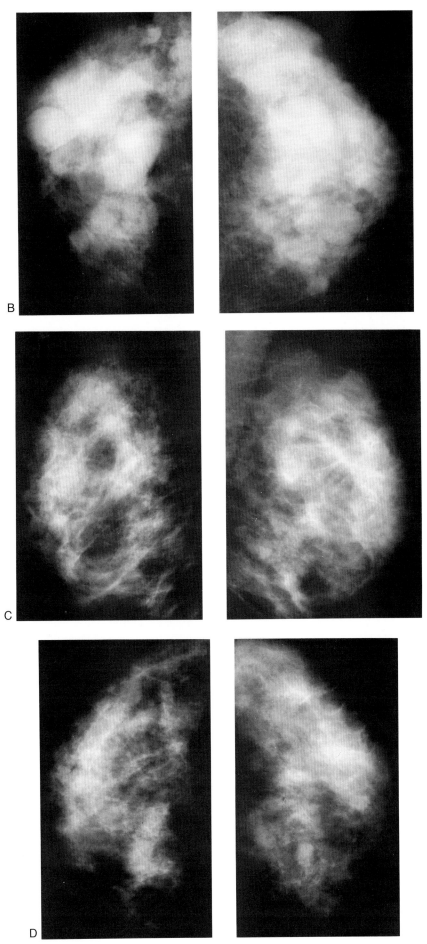

FIG. 13. (*Continued*)

ABSCESS DRAINAGE

Conventional treatment for breast abscesses is surgical incision and drainage under general anesthesia. Since breast abscesses occur most commonly in lactating women, a nonsurgical treatment would be invaluable. Ultrasound-guided percutaneous drainage can replace surgery in most cases (6). The procedure can easily be performed using only local anesthetic with the freehand technique described above. A 5 to 6 French "one-stick" trocar/catheter is guided toward the abscess under continuous ultrasound visualization (Fig. 14). The abscess is then punctured and drained quickly and easily. Occasionally, larger catheters may be necessary. Routine irrigation with saline breaks down septa and cleans the abscess cavity, which is periodically rechecked with ultrasound. After a few days, when the abscess cavity has resolved, the catheter can be removed, with excellent resultant cosmesis.

NEEDLE LOCALIZATION

Before the development of localization needles, nonpalpable lesions were localized externally. One method involved plotting lesion coordinates on a diagram of

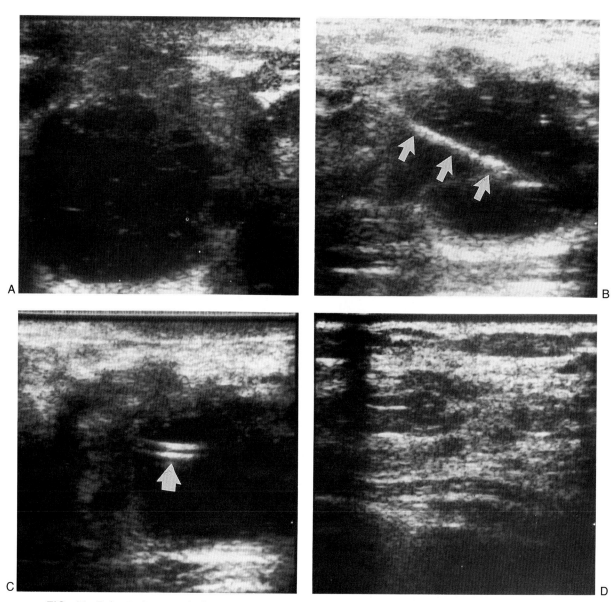

FIG. 14. Breast abscess drainage. **A:** Breast abscess visualized as a complex cystic mass on ultrasound. **B:** A 5 French one-stick trocar catheter advanced within the abscess (*arrows*). **C:** The trocar has been removed, and the catheter has coiled within the abscess (*arrow*). **D:** One week after ultrasound-guided abscess drainage, there is no evidence whatsoever of the previously drained abscess.

the breast that the surgeon used as a map. Another procedure included placing radiopaque markers on the skin overlying the lesion during mammography. Both of these techniques were imprecise and required excessive tissue removal (7).

Mammographically guided needle localization of breast lesions was developed to reduce the amount of tissue excised during biopsy (8–11). The original technique involved the freehand placement of a conventional 1½-inch hypodermic needle or a longer spinal needle in the breast, which the surgeon used as a guide to the lesion (8).

Although needle localization was more accurate than external localization, there were still significant problems with needle displacement before or during surgery. Several types of localization wires with hooked ends to secure the needle in place within the breast were developed to address this problem (7,12–16). Most radiologists now use one of a variety of hook wires for localization (Fig. 15).

With hook wires, lesions have traditionally been identified using standard mammography with or without a fenestrated compression plate. Most radiologists advocate placing the localizing wire within 1 cm of the

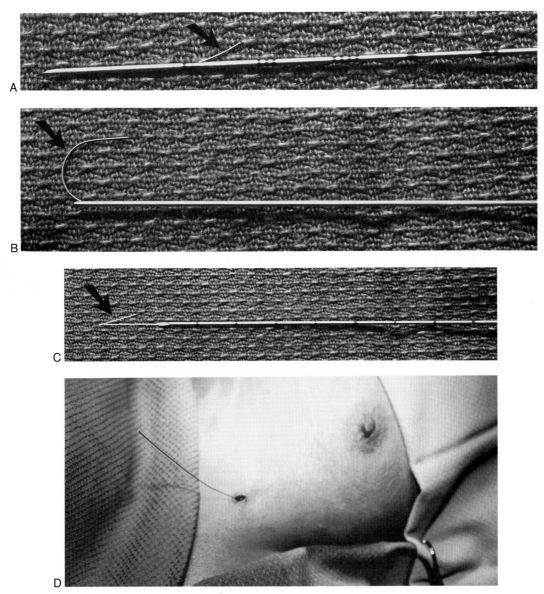

FIG. 15. Hook wire localization needles. **A:** Hawkins breast localization needle has a retractable sidewall barb (*arrow*) (National-Standard Medical Products, Gainesville, Florida) (*13*). **B:** Homer Mammolok needle has a retractable J-wire (*arrow*) (North American Instruments, Glen Falls, New York) (*14–16*). **C:** Kopans breast localization needle has a nonretractable hook wire (*arrow*) (Cook, Bloomington, Indiana) (*12*). **D:** Hook wire in place before surgical biopsy. (From Parker et al., Ref. 5a, with permission.)

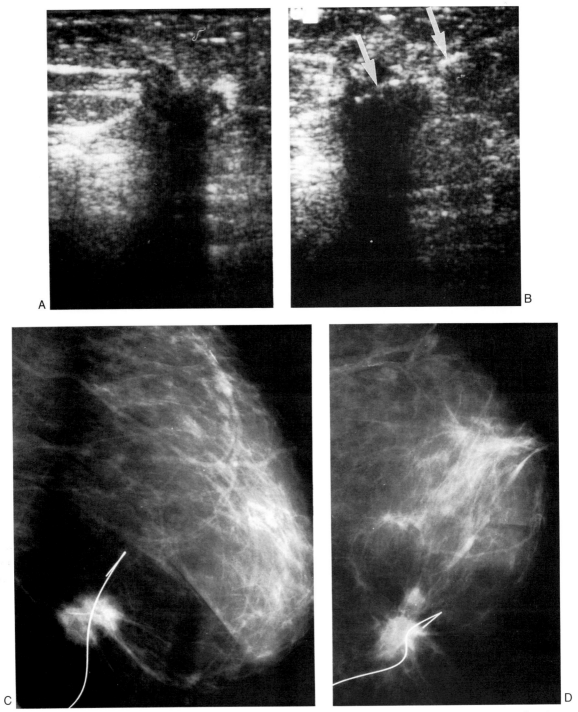

FIG. 16. Ultrasound-guided needle localization. **A:** Irregular hypoechoic lesion to be localized. **B:** Localization needle (*arrows*) coursing through the lesion. **C:** Mediolateral view of the final position of the hook wire after ultrasound localization. **D:** Craniocaudal view.

lesion (17–20). In practice, however, this is not always possible with mammography, and second attempts are necessary in a significant percentage of mammographic localizations. This occurs because mammography provides only two-dimensional ''snapshots in time.'' Le-

sion movement can occur between mammograms due to patient movement and/or breast retraction without the radiologist's knowledge. Also, the original oblique and craniocaudal mammogram views are not truly orthogonal, which makes it difficult to pinpoint the lesion in three dimensions. Finally, the position in which the mammographic localization is performed is different from the surgical position.

Large, pendulous breasts pose special problems in mammographic localization because they can assume many different positions in and out of compression, causing the lesion to appear to change location (9). Longer distances to lesions in large breasts can also create problems. The farther the needle has to travel to reach the lesion, the greater the likelihood of missing the target. When the needle is inserted into the breast at a slightly incorrect angle, even if the angle error remains constant, the farther the needle is advanced into the breast the farther off target the needle will end up. Even a small angle error can result in a significant distance error when localizing a deep lesion (see Figure 16 in Chapter 7).

Ultrasound has several advantages over mammography in guiding needle localization. First, the position in which the localization is performed is the same as the position for diagnostic breast ultrasound, which is similar to the surgical position. Second, with ultrasound, the needle and localization wire are visible in two planes in real time and the third plane is readily apparent with slight transducer movements. The exact relationship between the wire and the lesion is apparent (Fig. 16). Mobile lesions can be "chased down" under real-time control. Second attempts are virtually never necessary with ultrasound localizations because the wire is visible either through or immediately next to and touching the lesion.

Obviously, ultrasound localization is mandatory for lesions that are visible only by ultrasound. However, ultrasound localization is also possible for lesions that are both mammographically and ultrasonographically visible. At the BDCC all lesions that are seen with ultrasound are approached with ultrasound rather than mammographic guidance.

As with other breast interventions, ultrasound-guided needle and hook wire placement can be performed using the memory technique, a dedicated needle guide, or the freehand technique. Again, the freehand technique described above is the most accurate and flexible.

After the instillation of local anesthetic and under continuous real-time guidance, the needle is passed through the lesion if it is penetrable or immediately along the edge of the lesion if it is not (Fig. 16A,B). Either way, it is important to pass the needle *completely* through or beyond the lesion. The hook wire must open completely to lodge itself firmly in the breast but frequently cannot open within the denser tissue of the lesion itself.

Once the needle has been placed, 0.1 mL of methylene blue dye may be injected into the breast. Medicinal carbon also has been suggested as a marker because it does not diffuse through breast tissue (21). The hook wire is placed, and the needle is removed. Then the wire is scanned to confirm its position relative to the lesion. Since there is usually some air within the needle before dye is injected, small air bubbles are frequently sonographically visible along the needle path.

After ultrasound-guided wire placement, a unilateral mammogram is obtained. This is sent with the patient to surgery to help orient the surgeon (Fig. 16C,D). The skin directly over the terminus of the hook wire can be marked if the surgeon so desires.

Typically, postsurgical specimen radiography is not done on lesions localized with ultrasound. Of course, if the lesion is discrete and seen mammographically or contains microcalcifications, specimen radiography can be helpful.

CONCLUSION

Breast ultrasound is presently underutilized by most radiologists because there is some disagreement about its usefulness. However, the radiologists who feel or think that ultrasound should play only a minor role in breast imaging tend to be less familiar with ultrasound in general and use older equipment with suboptimal image quality. Those who are well trained in ultrasound and have state-of-the-art near-field imaging equipment use diagnostic breast ultrasound as an essential adjunct to mammography and clinical examination (22). Regardless of the debate over diagnostic breast ultrasound, however, there is no question that interventional breast ultrasound is an invaluable tool.

It is essential to assimilate the interventional techniques described in this chapter to gain mastery of ultrasound-guided large-core breast biopsy, which is described in the following chapter.

REFERENCES

1. Bassett LW, Kimme-Smith C. Breast sonography. *AJR Am J Roentgenol* 1991;156:449–455.
1a. Parker SH, Jobe WE, Dennis MA, et al. Ultrasound-guided automated large core breast biopsy. *Radiology* 1993;187:507–511.
2. Matalon TAS, Silver B. Ultrasound guidance of interventional procedures. *Radiology* 1990;174:43–47.
3. Dogliotti L, Orlandi F, Caraci P, et al. Biochemistry of breast cyst fluid. *Ann NY Acad Sci* 1990;586:17–28.
4. Bruzzi P, Bucchi L, Constantini M, Naldoni C. Biochemistry of breast cyst fluid: follow-up studies of patients with categorized breast cysts. *Ann NY Acad Sci* 1990;586:43–52.
5. Fornage BD. Fine-needle aspiration biopsy with a vacuum test tube. *Radiology* 1988;169:553–554.
5a. Parker SH, Jobe WE, Yakes WF. Breast intervention. In: Castaneda-Zuniga WF, ed. *Interventional Radiology*. 2nd ed. Baltimore: Williams & Wilkins, 1992;2:1291,1293.
6. Karstrup S, Nolsoe C, Brabrand K, Neilsen KR. Ultrasonically guided percutaneous drainage of breast abscesses. *Acta Radiol* 1990;31:157–159.

7. Feig SA. Methods and equipment for prebiopsy localization of nonpalpable breast lesions (syllabus). In Moskowitz M, ed. *A categorized course in diagnostic radiology breast imaging.* Presented at the 72nd Scientific Assembly and Annual Meeting for the Radiological Society of North America, Chicago, IL, Nov 30–Dec 5, 1986:53–60.
8. Dodd GD, Fry K, Delany W. Pre-op localization of occult carcinoma of the breast. In Nealon TF, ed. *Management of patients with cancer.* Philadelphia: WB Saunders, 1965:88–113.
9. Feig SA. Localization of clinically occult breast lesions. *Radiol Clin North Am* 1983;21:155–171.
10. Frank HA, Hall FM, Steer ML. Preoperative localization of nonpalpable breast lesions demonstrated by mammography. *N Engl J Med* 1976;295:259–260.
11. Threatt B, Apleman H, Dow R, et al. Percutaneous needle localization of clustered microcalcifications prior to biopsy. *Am J Roentgenol Radium Ther Nucl Med* 1974;121:839–842.
12. Meyer J, Kopans D, Stomper P, Lindfors K. Occult breast abnormalities: percutaneous pre-operative needle localization. *Radiology* 1984;150:335–337.
13. Urrutia EJ, Hawkins MC, Steinbach BG, et al. Retractable-barb needle for breast lesion localization: use in 60 cases. *Radiology* 1988;169:845–847.
14. Homer MJ. Nonpalpable breast lesion localization using a curved-end retractable wire. *Radiology* 1985;157:259–260.
15. Homer MJ, Pile-Spellman ER. Needle localization of occult breast lesions with a curved-end retractable wire: technique and pitfalls. *Radiology* 1986;161:547–548.
16. Homer MJ. Localization of nonpalpable breast lesions: technical aspects and analysis of 80 cases. *AJR Am J Roentgenol* 1985; 140:807–811.
17. Gallagher WJ, Cardenosa G, Rubens JR, et al. Minimal volume excision of nonpalpable breast lesions. *AJR Am J Roentgenol* 1989;153:957–961.
18. Gisvold JJ, Martin JK. Prebiopsy localization of nonpalpable breast lesions. *AJR Am J Roentgenol* 1984;143:477–481.
19. Bigelow R, Smith R, Goodman PA, Wilson GS. Needle localization of nonpalpable breast masses. *Arch Surg* 1985;120:565–569.
20. Tinnemans JGM, Wobbes T, Hendricks JHCL, et al. Localization and excision of nonpalpable breast lesions: a surgical evaluation of three methods. *Arch Surg* 1987;122:802–806.
21. Burhenne LW, Worth AJ, Burhenne HJ. Preoperative localization of nonpalpable breast lesions with medicinal carbon. Presented at the 76th Scientific Assembly and Annual Meeting of the Radiological Society of North America, Chicago, IL, Nov 25–30, 1990.
22. Fornage BD. Interventional ultrasound of the breast. In McGahan JP, ed. *Interventional ultrasound.* Baltimore: Williams & Wilkins; 1990:71–83.

Percutaneous Breast Biopsy, edited by
Steve H. Parker and William E. Jobe.
Raven Press, Ltd., New York © 1993.

CHAPTER 13

Ultrasound-guided Large-Core Breast Biopsy

Steve H. Parker and Mark A. Dennis

Although stereotactic mammography has proven extremely useful for identifying breast lesions, ultrasound opens up totally new avenues in the diagnosis and treatment of breast disease. Like stereotactic biopsy, ultrasound-guided core biopsy can be performed through an incision much smaller than that required for conventional excisional biopsy. However, ultrasound guidance has the additional advantage of continuous, real-time visualization. The ultrasound transducer becomes an extension of the senses, providing a "magic window" into the body. The radiologist integrates the movements of the transducer and needle so that he or she constantly views the appropriate region and the action taking place within it.

In many centers, mammographers, traditionally poorly versed in ultrasound and intervention, will be responsible for percutaneous breast biopsy (rather than interventionalists or ultrasonologists). To take full advantage of ultrasound's potential, however, mammographers will need to become more conversant with both ultrasound and interventional techniques. In practices where interventionalists or ultrasonologists perform breast biopsy, they will need to become more knowledgeable about breast disease. Since percutaneous breast biopsy is most effective when both ultrasound and stereotactic guidance are available, it is probably better for the same radiologist to be responsible for breast biopsy regardless of the imaging technique used. Dividing this responsibility among ultrasonologists, mammographers, and interventionalists on the basis of equipment dilutes the experience of each physician. Such division can also confuse ordering physicians and their patients, as well as complicate patient flow. (For a detailed description of patient selection and workup, see Chapter 7.)

S.H. Parker and M.A. Dennis: Radiology Imaging Associates, Breast Diagnostic and Counseling Centre, Englewood, Colorado 80111.

GUIDANCE SELECTION

Each patient with mammographic or clinical findings that might require biopsy should be evaluated with breast ultrasound to select the appropriate imaging technique (mammography or ultrasound) for the biopsy. Most cases of microcalcifications are the only exception. Naturally, if the abnormality includes mammographic microcalcifications without an associated mass or density, the likelihood of locating the abnormality on ultrasound is small. In these cases, diagnostic ultrasound examination generally is not warranted. Diagnostic ultrasound also may not be indicated when the radiologist is not comfortable with ultrasound and does not intend to guide the biopsy with it. On the other hand, when ultrasound guidance is an option, scanning for microcalcifications in patients who cannot tolerate the positioning required for stereotactic biopsy can still sometimes prove fruitful (Fig. 1).

At the Breast Diagnostic and Counseling Centre, any abnormality that can be seen with breast ultrasound is biopsied with ultrasound guidance because this method has certain advantages over stereotactic breast biopsy. First, ultrasound does not use ionizing radiation. Although the amount of radiation involved in a stereotactic biopsy is quite small, it is prudent to avoid exposure whenever possible. Second, the procedure can be performed much more quickly with ultrasound guidance compared with stereotaxis. Less time is involved in both patient positioning and filming. Finally, the patient is generally more comfortable in the supine position rather than the prone position and the breast is not in compression.

PREBIOPSY PROCEDURES

With a good team approach, the radiologist does not need to be present until the patient has been posi-

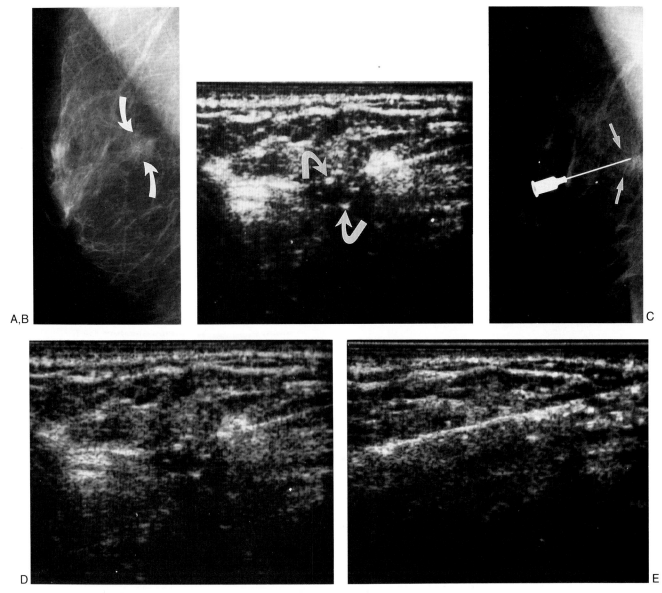

FIG. 1. Ultrasound-guided biopsy of microcalcifications in an arthritic patient who was intolerant of stereotactic positioning. **A:** Mediolateral view showing a cluster of calcifications (*curved arrows*) with associated density. **B:** Ultrasound interrogation of the region revealed a number of punctate echogenicities (*curved arrows*) thought to represent the calcifications. The hypoechoic region surrounding the echogenicities was thought to correspond to the mammographic density. **C:** A quick, ultrasound-guided needle localization was performed with a 25 gauge hypodermic needle (*arrows*). **D:** Repeat mediolateral view after needle localization proved that the ultrasound finding was the microcalcifications. **E:** Core biopsy was then performed using ultrasound instead of stereotactic guidance. The histologic diagnosis was infiltrating ductal carcinoma.

tioned, prepared, and draped. By conferring with the radiologist regarding the patient and the diagnostic workup ahead of time, the technologist and nurse can usually handle all of the patient preparation while the radiologist attends to other patients and/or duties (see Chapters 4 and 5).

Generally, the BDCC nurse performs most of the counseling, and the radiologist gets involved only at the patient's request. Some radiologists may prefer to counsel the patients themselves. Regardless of who

counsels the patient, it is imperative to educate her as completely as possible. Patients at the BDCC are informed that stereotactic biopsy may also be necessary to evaluate this or other lesions. Rebiopsy or surgical excision could also be recommended. It should be emphasized to the patient that no biopsy method, including surgery, is perfect. The importance of follow-up, both clinical and radiologic, should also be stressed.

Before the biopsy, the radiologist confers with the

technologist about the case to finalize the appropriate set up. With proper training, the technologist can make and implement most of the set-up decisions without the radiologist's input. In this prebiopsy conference the location and number of lesions are confirmed. All clinical and mammographic concerns should be discussed so that there is no confusion in the patient's presence.

The possibility of prebiopsy aspiration is also discussed. As noted earlier, attempted aspiration can differentiate among solid, complex, and cystic lesions (see Chapter 12). When the patient and equipment have been properly prepared, proceeding directly to ultra-

sound-guided core biopsy of lesions that cannot be aspirated is quite easy. Naturally, if a lesion turns out to be a complex cyst that is aspirated completely, no core biopsy is necessary. If any solid component remains after aspiration of some of the contents, core biopsy is indicated (see Fig. 7 in Chapter 12).

If there is any question about whether an ultrasound lesion corresponds to a given mammographic lesion, an ultrasound-guided needle localization can be performed quickly and easily (Fig. 2). A 25 gauge hypodermic needle is placed in the ultrasound lesion under continuous ultrasound guidance. A mammogram documenting the needle's location within the breast is then

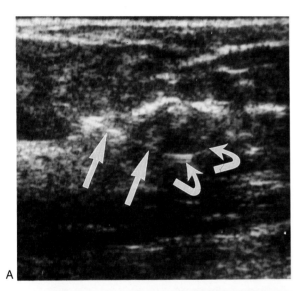

FIG. 2. Ultrasound-guided needle localization with a retractable hook wire system performed before core biopsy. **A:** Ultrasound showing the distal end of the needle (**arrows**) within the center of the lesion. The extruded, retractable J-wire (*curved arrows*) curves anteriorly toward the transducer. **B:** Postlocalization mediolateral mammogram. When viewed with Fig. 2C, this mammogram confirms that the ultrasonographic and mammographic lesions are the same. **C:** Postlocalization craniocaudal mammography. When viewed with Fig. 2B, this confirms that the ultrasonographic and mammographic lesions are the same. After the confirmatory mammogram was performed, the wire was retracted and the needle was removed before ultrasound-guided core biopsy was performed.

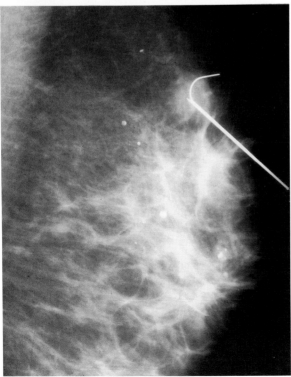

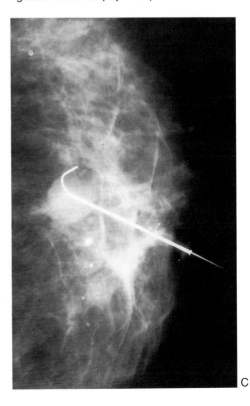

compared to the original mammogram. Occasionally, the hypodermic needle is dislodged from its original position during mammographic positioning and compression. If displacement is suspected, the breast can be reexamined with ultrasound to determine whether the needle is still within the ultrasonographic lesion. If the needle has moved and it is still not clear whether the mammographic and ultrasonographic lesions are the same, the localization can be repeated with a retractable hook wire. Alternatively, the localization can be performed at the outset with a retractable-wire needle, although these are more expensive than the standard hypodermic needles. After confirming that the ultrasound and mammographic lesions are the same, the radiologist can retract the wire and remove the needle. If localization identifies two separate lesions, one visualized only mammographically and one visualized only ultrasonographically, then each lesion can be biopsied separately—with one biopsy using stereotaxis and one using ultrasound for guidance.

EQUIPMENT

As with diagnostic and interventional breast ultrasound, the ultrasound equipment used in ultrasound-guided core biopsy is critical to the success of the procedure. Many manufacturers make ultrasound equipment that can be used for breast ultrasound. It has been erroneously stated, however, that any low-cost ultrasound equipment would be adequate (1). As noted earlier, the equipment must be state of the art with high-frequency (7.5 to 10.0 mHz), electronically focused, linear array transducers capable of producing excellent near-field images (see Chapter 10). The transducer also should be compact and light. Price alone does not ensure high-quality near-field imaging, since some machines costing over $200,000 are still not adequate for good breast ultrasound (Fig. 3). Equipment must be evaluated on an image rather than a price basis.

Frequently, old, outdated ultrasound equipment is retired from the general ultrasound section to the breast section, probably because of a lack of ultrasound experience on the part of the radiologists responsible for breast imaging. Unfortunately, however, state-of-the-art equipment is essential in breast imaging. Using suboptimal equipment in the breast where image quality is critical creates a never-ending cycle. Inexperienced radiologists who do not have access to the kind of equipment that would allow them to improve their skills are unable to recognize that better equipment is necessary. When economy is a consideration, older ultrasound equipment that provides adequate images of deeper, larger organs such as the gallbladder and uterus can continue to be used in that capacity. However, these machines do not provide the high-resolution, near-field images needed to evaluate the comparatively smaller, more superficial lesions in the breast. Good breast ultrasound is virtually impossible without state-of-the-art equipment.

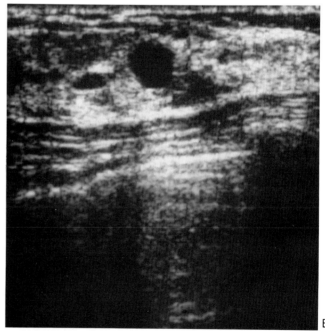

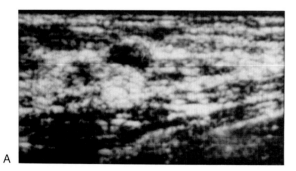

FIG. 3. Comparison of ultrasound equipment. **A:** Two hypoechoic lesions identified with a nationally known ultrasound unit in a patient referred to the BDCC for biopsy. **B:** AI 5200 image of same lesions clearly demonstrating that they are simple cysts. Therefore, no biopsy was performed.

TECHNIQUE

Details of the entire procedure from the nurse's, technologist's, and radiation physicist's points of view are discussed in Chapters 4, 5, and 6, respectively. Core biopsy with stereotactic guidance is covered in Chapter 7.

Generally, it is most convenient to position the ultrasound machine near the patient's head on the same side as the involved breast. This eliminates the passing of a nonsterile transducer cord across the patient's body and the potential contamination of the biopsy field. The radiologist will be most comfortable seated in the "V" formed by the ultrasound machine and the procedure table (Fig. 4). Here the radiologist can look back and forth at the ultrasound screen, the transducer and needle, and the patient's breast without significantly changing body or head position.

Once the patient, radiologist, technologist, and nurse are comfortable, the procedure can begin. The first step, of course, is sterile scanning of the breast to localize the lesion. Orienting the needle under the long axis of the transducer allows the radiologist to visualize the entire length of the needle rather than just the needle tip (Fig. 5). Radiologists new to ultrasound-guided core breast biopsy may prefer to scan the breast in a nonsterile fashion before it is prepped and draped. Decisions can then be made about how to approach the lesion without the encumbrances of sterile technique. Marking the desired skin entry point with an indelible marker or imprinting the skin with a retracted ballpoint

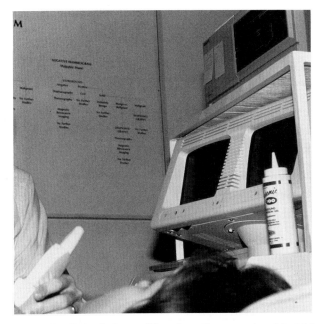

FIG. 4. Radiologist's position for ultrasound-guided biopsy. When positioned between the ultrasound equipment and the patient, the radiologist can glance between the two quite easily.

pen allows radiologists to reorient themselves quickly after the breast is sterile (Fig. 6).

Either way, after locating the lesion the radiologist plans the appropriate route to the lesion. Several factors should be considered, including the depth of the lesion, the angle of the chest wall, and the presence and amount of dense fibrous tissue in the vicinity of the lesion. The depth of the lesion influences the angle of approach. From a technical standpoint, superficial lesions are generally the easiest to biopsy. Superficial lesions can be approached more parallel to the transducer than can deeper lesions, while still maintaining a relatively direct route (see Fig. 5A in Chapter 12). Deeper lesions require a less parallel, more oblique approach, which makes it more difficult to visualize the needle. Normally, the transducer is positioned with the lesion in the center of the image. With deep lesions, however, the transducer is positioned with the lesion to one side of the image (i.e., the lesion is visualized on one end of the transducer and the needle entry point is visualized on the other) (see Fig. 5B in Chapter 12). In this way the course of the needle will be as close to parallel as possible, ensuring the best needle visualization. As the periphery of the lesion is approached, the needle can be levered downward. This compresses the outer portion of the breast and brings the needle more parallel to the transducer, further enhancing needle visualization (see Fig. 6A in Chapter 12). Thus, deeper lesions require a skin entry point slightly further from the lesion so that the needle can move as closely as possible in a horizontal course.

Lesions close to or abutting the chest wall can be biopsied with ultrasound guidance but pose some additional problems that require alteration of the biopsy approach. With appropriate planning, however, chest wall lesions can be approached confidently and safely.

One way to approach chest wall lesions would be to move the skin entry point well away from the lesion so that a course more parallel to the chest wall is assumed (see Fig. 6B in Chapter 12). This approach has two drawbacks, however. First, the farther the skin entry point is from the transducer, the harder it is to observe the needle and keep it in the plane of the ultrasound beam. Second, this approach generally places the skin entry point considerably farther from the lesion than does the more direct oblique approach. Some surgeons excise the needle tract during lumpectomy. If the lesion turns out to be cancer and lumpectomy is performed, more tissue is excised than if a more direct oblique approach had created a shorter needle tract.

Thus, for most chest wall lesions, the oblique approach used for other deep lesions is preferable. Since the needle enters the skin at a relatively steep angle, as close to the transducer as possible, a medial to lateral (rather than lateral to medial) approach takes advantage of the chest wall's natural curvature. Again, this

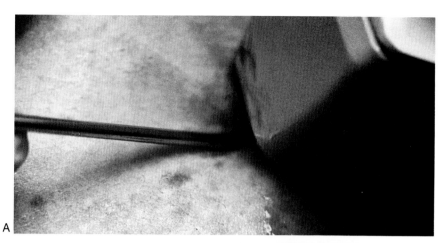

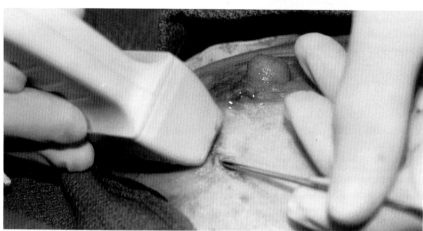

FIG. 5. Proper orientation of the needle relative to the transducer. **A:** The needle enters the skin at the margin of the transducer and is advanced under the long axis. Maintaining the needle's physical position in the center of the transducer keeps the needle in the center of the ultrasound beam as well. **B:** A common mistake with ultrasound guidance is not maintaining the needle in the center of the transducer. In this case, a quick glance down at the hands would reveal why the needle was not imaged on the screen.

involves positioning of the transducer with the lesion on one side and the skin entry point on the other. Instilling local anesthetic into the region between the lesion and the chest wall can raise the lesion somewhat. Then, by introducing the biopsy needle into the space between the lesion and chest wall and levering it downward, one compresses the underlying breast tissue along the shaft of the needle. This creates an approach that avoids the chest wall (see Fig. 6A in Chapter 12 and Fig. 7 in this chapter).

When lesions are surrounded by a considerable amount of dense fibrous tissue, it is important to plan an approach that avoids this tissue if possible. (The same applies to ultrasound-guided needle localizations; see Chapter 12.) There are two reasons for this. First, dense fibrous tissue tends to be the most sensitive tissue within the breast, especially in younger women. Even 25 gauge aspiration or anesthetic needles can elicit marked discomfort when this tissue is traversed.

Second, it can be very difficult to penetrate these areas with any sort of needle. If no alternative route is available and dense fibrous tissue must be traversed, liberal instillation of local anesthetic is imperative. Although considerable force may be required to advance the 14 gauge needle through dense fibrous tissue manually, firing the Biopty gun into this tissue can aid in establishing a tract. A potential problem arises, however, when a different area of the lesion needs to be sampled. Since the needle is confined to the course of the needle tract, it may be difficult to change the angle of approach. If this occurs, it may be necessary to establish several different tracts to canvass the lesion completely.

When choosing a skin entry point, the possibility of breast conservation surgery should always be kept in mind as well, especially when the lesion is highly suspicious for cancer yet small enough to permit lumpectomy. As mentioned earlier, many surgeons prefer to excise the needle tract at the time of lumpectomy. The location of the needle tract thus can alter the surgeon's approach to the lumpectomy. When possible, many surgeons prefer a periareolar approach that blends the incision into the border between the areola and the breast because it creates a better cosmetic result. A skin entry point (for core biopsy) approximately 1 cm from the areolar margin allows excision of the needle tract so that the skin margins are at the border of the areola. Other surgeons want the radiologist to use a skin entry point along the radial line equidistant from the areola. Every surgeon's approach to lumpectomy and needle tract excision is at least slightly different. Therefore, it is prudent for radiologists to familiarize themselves with the local surgical community's and referring surgeons' standards so that the appropriate skin entry point can be selected.

After the skin entry point and route to the lesion are selected, the skin is anesthetized with a ⅝-inch 25 to 30 gauge anesthetic needle. Alternatively, an anesthetic spray or an automated anesthetic administrator can be used. After this, a longer 1¼-inch 25 gauge needle is used to administer deeper local anesthetic along the projected path of the biopsy needle and around the lesion (Fig. 8). Occasionally, a longer 22 gauge spinal needle may be required to reach a very deep lesion in a large breast. Since it requires only a short time to administer and, unlike with stereotactic biopsy, does

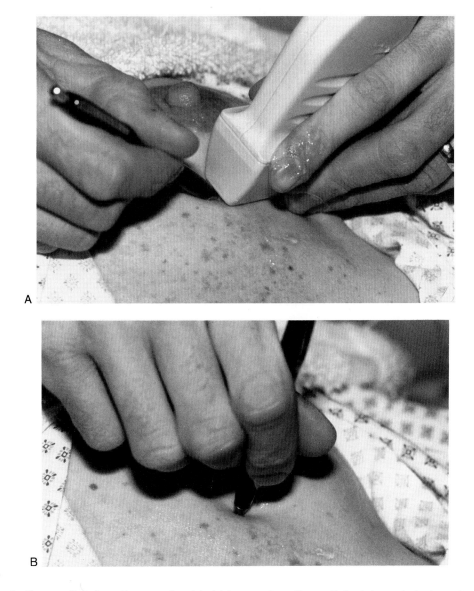

FIG. 6. Preparation for ultrasound-guided biopsy when the radiologist needs to be oriented to the biopsy approach before the breast is prepared and draped. **A:** A ballpoint pen with the point retracted can be used to simulate the planned approach with the needle. **B:** Once the desired skin entry point is chosen, an indentation made with the pen will not wash off when the breast is prepped.

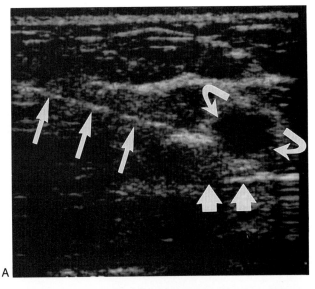

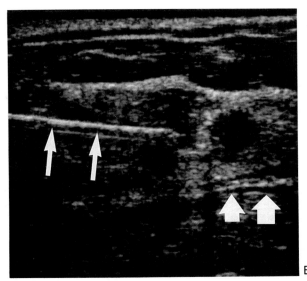

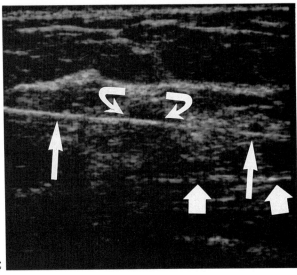

FIG. 7. Approaching a chest wall lesion. **A:** The needle (*long arrows*) is directed into the space between the chest wall (*short arrows*) and the lesion (*curved arrows*). **B:** The needle (*long arrows*) is then levered down until it is nearly parallel to the chest wall (*short arrows*). **C:** The postfire view shows that the needle (*long arrows*) has coursed through the lesion (*curved arrows*) while avoiding the chest wall (*short arrows*). (From Parker et al., Ref. 5, with permission.)

not potentially obscure visualization of the lesion, deep local anesthetic is strongly recommended in every patient to eliminate any possibility for pain. As long as the anesthetic is mixed with sodium bicarbonate, the patient should feel virtually nothing during its administration, as well as during the biopsy (see Chapters 4 and 7).

After liberally anesthetizing the breast, the operator makes a small skin nick with a scalpel (Fig. 9). This nick need only be large enough to admit the 14 gauge needle easily through the skin. The resultant defect is not really larger than if the skin were pierced directly with the 14 gauge needle. Although extremely sharp needles can pierce the skin *de novo*, skin resistance along the outer cannula retards its rapid action and produces a suboptimal sample. Without a skin nick,

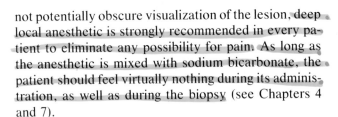

FIG. 8. Instillation of local anesthetic. **A:** The needle courses under the long axis of the transducer in the same way as it does during other ultrasound-guided procedures. **B:** Ultrasound image of the 25 gauge anesthetic needle (*straight arrows*) at the anterior margin of the lesion (*curved arrows*). **C:** Hypoechoic anesthetic (*short arrows*) is seen being deposited around the periphery of the lesion (*curved arrows*). **D:** The first needle core pass (*arrows*) through the lesion elicited some discomfort. (From Parker et al., Ref. *1a*, with permission.) **E:** Therefore, more anesthetic (*arrow*) was placed on the back side of the lesion before additional passes. Subsequent passes were then performed without discomfort.

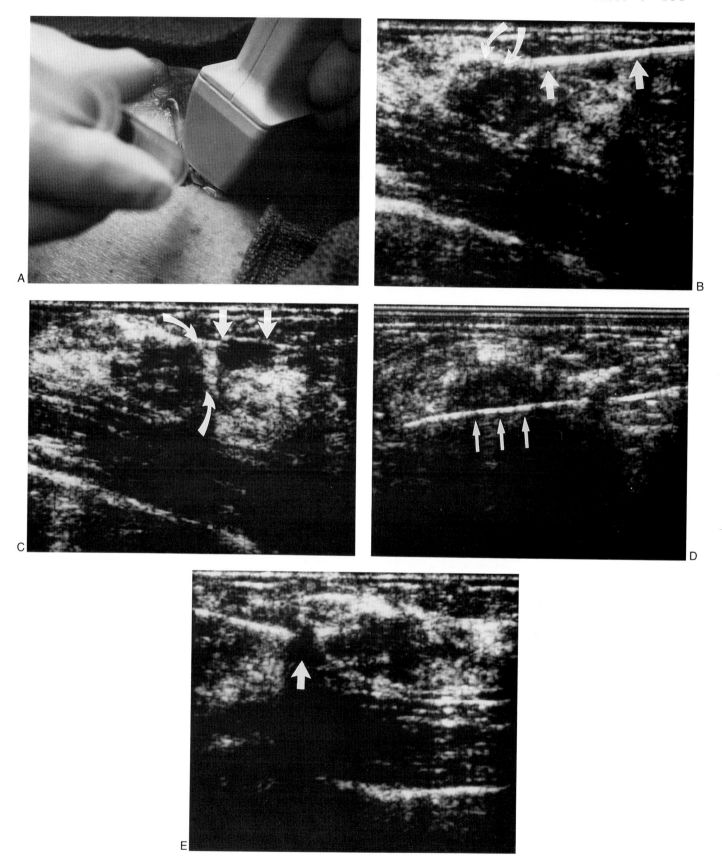

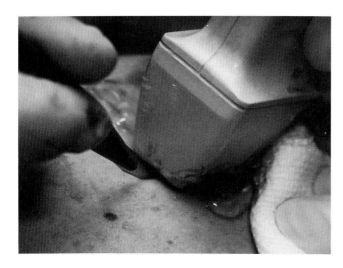

FIG. 9. Small skin nick made with the scalpel at the desired skin entry point after the administration of anesthetic.

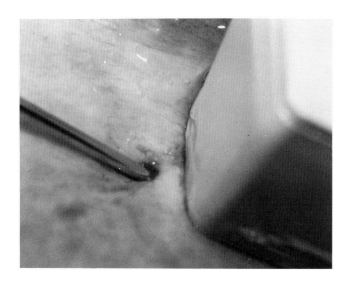

FIG. 10. Under continuous ultrasound monitoring, the needle is guided through the nick with ease.

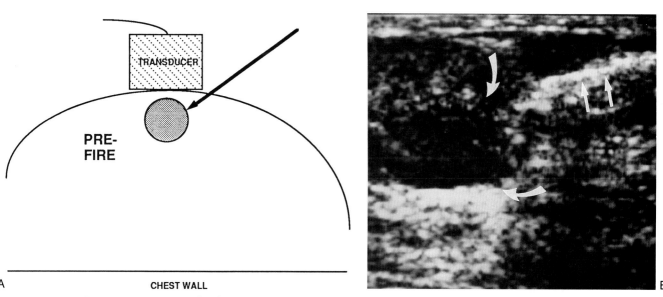

TRANSDUCER

PRE-FIRE

CHEST WALL

A   B

FIG. 11. Pre- and postfire images of ultrasound-guided biopsy. **A:** Schematic representation of the needle in the prefire position at the periphery of the lesion. **B:** Prefire ultrasound image showing the needle (*straight arrows*) poised at the periphery of the lesion (*curved arrows*).

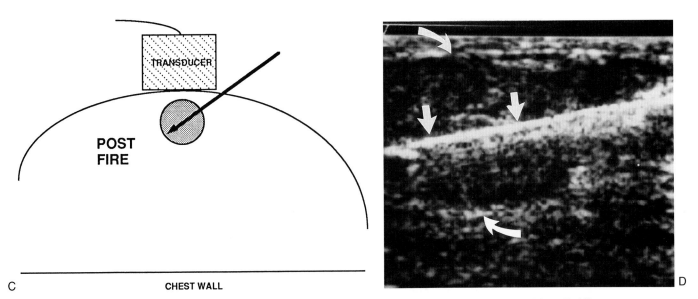

FIG. 11. (*Continued*) **C:** Schematic representation of the needle in the postfire position. **D:** Ultrasound image of the needle (*straight arrows*) in the postfire position coursing through the lesion (*curved arrows*). (From Parker et al., Ref. *5,* with permission.)

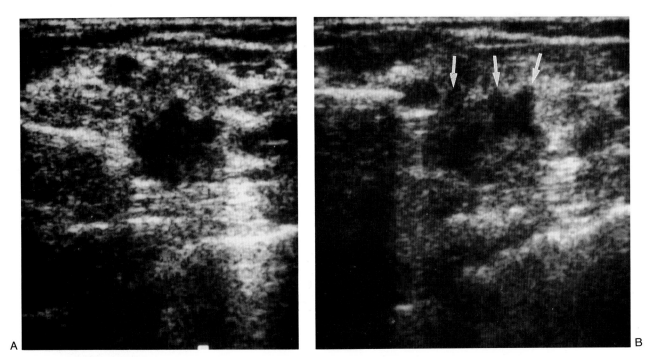

FIG. 12. Ultrasound-guided biopsy of an infiltrating ductal carcinoma with an intraductal component. **A:** Prefire ultrasound image of a lesion histologically diagnosed as infiltrating ductal carcinoma. **B:** Prefire ultrasound image of the biopsy of the hypoechoic "fingers" (*arrows*) projecting from the main lesion, which contained the intraductal component.

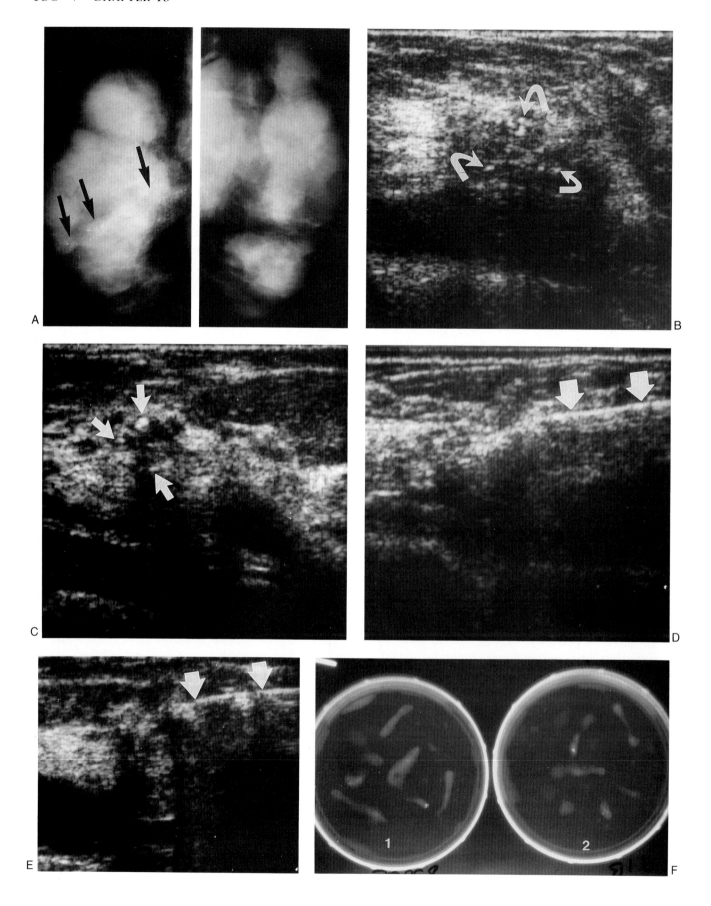

several passes are required before the resistance is eliminated. It is helpful, as well, to wiggle the tip of the scalpel back and forth just inside the skin when making the nick. This helps break up the subcutaneous tissues, again allowing easier passage of the needle and unrestricted, rapid action of the outer cannula.

Next, with the transducer in one hand and the needle in the other, the radiologist guides the needle through the skin nick and toward the lesion under continuous ultrasound visualization (Fig. 10). When the Biopty gun is used, a nonsterile assistant stabilizes the handle while the radiologist grasps the shaft of the needle to guide it. The nonsterile assistant keeps the handle in line with the needle while the radiologist changes its angle and depth. Completely sterile and disposable 14 gauge biopsy guns would give the radiologist total control over both the needle and the handle. These are not yet available, however.

Once the needle arrives at the periphery of the lesion, a prefire image is obtained (Fig. 11A,B). The gun is then fired, and a postfire image documents the needle coursing through the lesion (Fig. 11C,D). As with stereotactic breast biopsy, a minimum of five passes is recommended: one pass through the center of the lesion followed by one pass each through the anterior, posterior, craniad, and caudad portions of the lesion. The four peripheral passes generally sample generous portions of the lesion's margins. If intraductal extension of the lesion is suspected ultrasonographically, it should be investigated by biopsy through the involved ducts as well as the main body of the lesion (Fig. 12).

The samples are handled in the same way as those obtained with stereotactic biopsy. All samples from the same lesion are placed in one sterile specimen cup with a small amount of physiologic saline. Once samples from each lesion are collected, 10% formalin is added to fix the core tissue. If microcalcifications are associated with the ultrasonographic lesion, a specimen radiograph can be performed before the addition of the formalin (Fig. 13) (see Chapter 5). Naturally, each pathologist who reads core specimens may want the radiologist to adjust specimen handling to meet the protocol of the particular laboratory. Again, as with surgical standards, pathologic standards should be established jointly.

After the biopsy, manual pressure is held over the

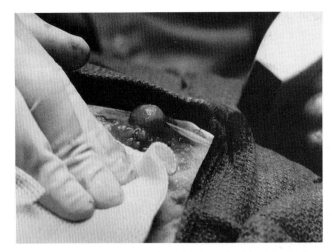

FIG. 14. Manual pressure is held over the biopsy site between passes (and for at least five minutes after the last pass).

biopsy site, including the needle tract and the lesion, for at least five minutes (Fig. 14). Prolonged oozing of blood during the biopsy naturally indicates longer compression. A compression bandage is then applied to the breast. (For complete details of postbiopsy care and counseling, see Chapter 4).

The patient returns on the following day to be reexamined. Although some radiologists may prefer to assume all responsibility for follow-up examination, an experienced nurse can perform these duties, freeing the radiologist to answer questions only at the patient's request. Either way, if any clinical concern arises, an ultrasound examination can rule out hematoma. It is inappropriate to assume that a hematoma exists on the basis of physical examination alone. Ultrasound has demonstrated that virtually all cases of postbiopsy "lump" at the BDCC were edematous breast tissue without a discrete mass or fluid collection (i.e., not hematomas). Ecchymosis and some interstitial bleeding are not uncommon, however. In addition, no significant infection or other complication has been reported by radiologists using this procedure (2–4).

If no problems are encountered on the follow-up clinical visit, the patient is advised to resume normal activities. Patients at the BDCC return in six months for a follow-up ultrasound examination and a unilateral mammogram to ensure that there has been no change.

FIG. 13. Ultrasound-guided biopsy of microcalcifications. **A:** Mammogram showing extremely dense breasts with calcifications (*arrows*) extending from the right subareolar region to the chest wall. **B:** Ultrasound of the deep right breast revealed multiple punctate echogenicities within a hypoechoic background (*curved arrows*). **C:** Ultrasound of the superficial periareolar region likewise revealed echogenicities (*short arrows*) thought to represent calcifications. **D:** Prefire view of the needle (*arrowheads*) approaching the deep lesion. **E:** Prefire view of the needle (*arrowheads*) approaching the superficial periareolar lesion. **F:** Specimen radiograph of cores from both regions (*1,* deep lesion; *2,* superficial lesion) demonstrates multiple calcifications in both. The histologic diagnosis was DCIS in both cases.

Some radiologists use a 4-month follow-up regimen, and some will undoubtedly recommend a 12-month follow-up. Regardless of the interval, if the findings remain stable at follow-up and continue to fit the needle core diagnosis, the patient can return to routine screening.

THE TEAM APPROACH

After the biopsy team gains extensive experience, the radiologist's participation can be limited to the actual biopsy passes themselves. Pre- and postbiopsy details can be handled by the rest of the biopsy team. A typical uncomplicated ultrasound-guided needle core biopsy of the breast can consume as little as five to ten minutes of the radiologist's time. As with stereotactic biopsies, ultrasound biopsies are scheduled one hour apart. This allows enough time to finalize the prebiopsy workup; counsel, position, and prepare the patient; perform the biopsy and postbiopsy care; review postbiopsy instructions; clean the biopsy room and apparatus; set up a new biopsy tray; and prepare the room for the next patient.

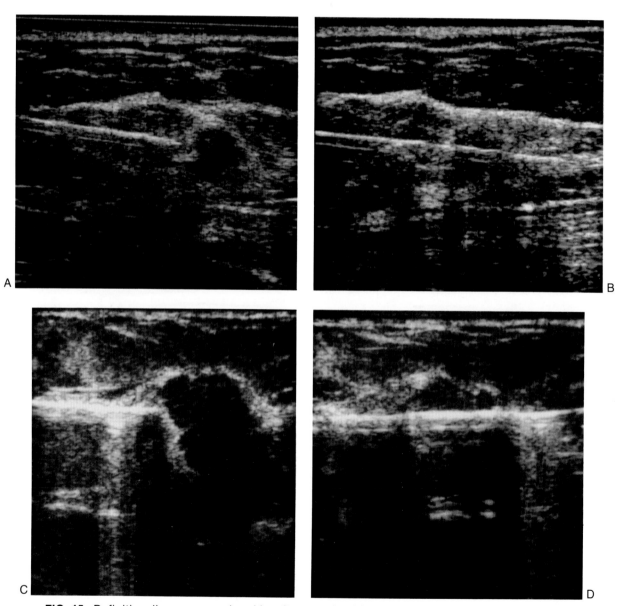

FIG. 15. Definitive diagnoses rendered by ultrasound-guided biopsy. **A:** Prefire view of a biopsy of a fibroadenoma. **B:** Postfire view of a biopsy of a fibroadenoma. **C:** Prefire view of an infiltrating ductal carcinoma. **D:** Postfire view of an infiltrating ductal carcinoma.

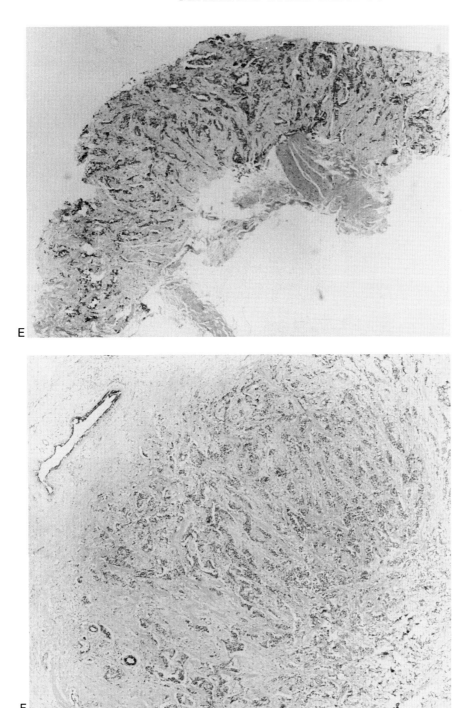

FIG. 15. (*Continued*) **E:** Core biopsy specimen showing infiltrating ductal carcinoma. **F:** Surgical specimen showing the exact same architecture as in the core specimen. (From Parker et al., Ref. *5,* with permission.)

CONCLUSION

Real-time ultrasound provides continuous visualization during biopsy. With automated large-gauge needles, this technique renders definitive histologic diagnoses with an accuracy equivalent to that of surgical diagnosis (Fig. 15) (5). Patient selection is similar to that for surgical biopsy. Additionally, lower suspicion cases can also be included when the patient's anxiety or physician's suspicion is significant. Proper breast imaging workup must be performed before biopsy. Dogged pursuit of the lesion and postfire images documenting the needle traversing the lesion are of paramount importance. It is also imperative that tissue samples be of superior quality and quantity. Only when both accurate needle placement and adequate tissue

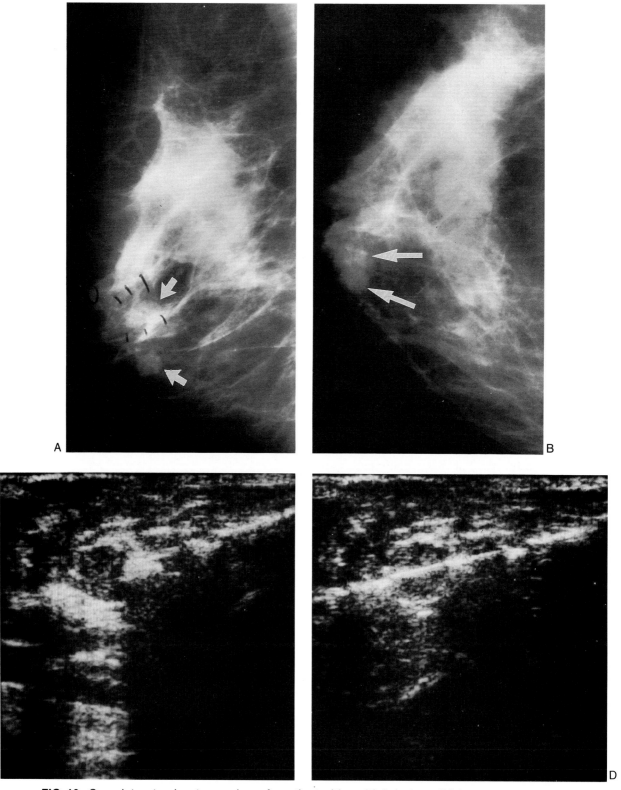

FIG. 16. Complete, step-by-step workup of a patient with multiple lesions. With proper ultrasound interrogation followed by ultrasound core biopsy of the solid lesions, this patient's three breast lesions were diagnosed in one visit. **A:** Mediolateral mammogram revealing at least two lesions (*arrows*) in the 6 o'clock position of the breast. **B:** Craniocaudal mammogram revealing at least two lesions (*arrows*) in the 6 o'clock position of the breast. The more superior lesion was noted to be a simple cyst on ultrasound, and therefore no further investigation of this lesion was deemed necessary. The more inferior lesion was noted to be solid, however. In addition, a second solid lesion was found in the 12 o'clock position of the breast. **C:** Prefire view of the core biopsy of the 6 o'clock lesion, which was histologically diagnosed as a fibroadenoma. **D:** Postfire view of the core biopsy of the 6 o'clock lesion, which was histologically diagnosed as a fibroadenoma.

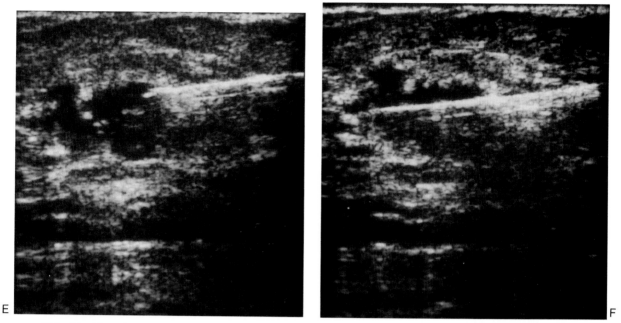

FIG. 16. (*Continued*) **E:** Prefire view of the core biopsy of the 12 o'clock lesion histologically diagnosed as infiltrating ductal carcinoma. **F:** Postfire view of the core biopsy of the 12 o'clock lesion, histologically diagnosed as infiltrating ductal carcinoma.

harvest have been assured can the radiologist consider the biopsy successful. If all of these requirements are met, ultrasound-guided breast biopsy can be an expedient, cost-effective, and dependable alternative to surgical biopsy (Fig. 16).

REFERENCES

1. Bassett LW, Kimme-Smith C. Breast sonography. *AJR Am J Roentgenol* 1991;156:449–455.
1a. Parker SH, Jobe WE, Yakes WF. Breast intervention. In: Castaneda-Zuniga WF, ed. *Interventional Radiology*. 2nd ed. Baltimore: Williams & Wilkins, 1992;2:1307.
2. Charboneau JW, Reading CC, Welch TJ. CT and sonographically guided needle biopsy: current techniques and new innovations. *AJR Am J Roentgenol* 1990;154:1–10.
3. Myer JE. Value of large-core biopsy of occult breast lesions. *AJR Am J Roentgenol* 1992;158:991–992.
4. Dronkers DJ. Stereotaxic core biopsy of breast lesions. *Radiology* 1992;183:631–634.
5. Parker SH, Jobe WE, Dennis MA, et al. Ultrasound-guided automated large core breast biopsy. *Radiology* [*in press*].

Percutaneous Breast Biopsy, edited by
Steve H. Parker and William E. Jobe.
Raven Press, Ltd., New York © 1993.

CHAPTER 14

Recent and Future Developments

Steve H. Parker and R. Edward Hendrick

A vast role awaits the radiologist in the diagnosis and treatment of breast disease. The ability to direct a biopsy needle with precision into breast lesions is only the beginning. New developments in the guidance techniques for breast biopsy will lead to new interventional applications. Presurgical, image-guided axillary lymph node biopsy could alter breast cancer workup and treatment. With continuing improvement in stereotactic mammography and ultrasound equipment, needle-borne tumor ablation may become possible. Improved MRI techniques, particularly with dedicated breast coils or even dedicated MRI mammography equipment, will enhance the role of MRI in breast disease. Radiologists who want to make full use of these technological advances will need to expand their expertise to include mammography, ultrasound, MRI, and interventional techniques.

MAMMOGRAPHY

Further refinements of the recumbent stereotactic table will provide better breast access and patient comfort. A number of improvements are being considered (e.g., a thinner table, a more pliable material for the breast aperture, and articulations in the table where the patient's head rests).

The possibility of human error in transferring computer-generated lesion coordinates to the biopsy unit itself is being addressed. Already automatic servo-mechanical entry optionally replaces manual entry of horizontal and vertical coordinates. A system designed to allow the computer to communicate directly with the needle-alignment device further decreases operator error by automatically aligning the biopsy needle (Fig. 1). The operator can then manually insert the needle to the specified depth coordinate.

An "auto-guide" system has been used at the Breast Diagnostic and Counseling Center in the following manner. When the center of the lesion is digitized, the other four peripheral targets are automatically placed in memory. With the push of a button, the needle carriage moves to the appropriate position. Pre- and postfire views of the biopsy of the lesion's center are then obtained. The radiologist biopsies the remaining four points while the pre- and postfire films are being developed. By the time those films are processed, the four remaining biopsies have already been completed. If the targeting was proven accurate, the procedure is ended. This method reduces the entire biopsy procedure to the time required to obtain and develop the pre- and postfire stereo views.

Thus far, in about 20% of cases biopsied with this method, retargeting and further biopsy have been necessary. Again, with the "auto-guide" this is much quicker than if the targeting were done manually. When retargeting is necessary, the cores obtained on the first targeting are still sent for histologic analysis. Naturally, this provides an even better indication of the surrounding breast milieu.

The most recent and exciting development in stereotactic mammography is the charged coupled device, which virtually instantaneously displays digitized images on a computer monitor (Fig. 2). The exquisite resolution of these images may surpass traditional screen-film mammography, with much less radiation. Nearly immediate image acquisition will considerably shorten the biopsy, thereby decreasing patient discomfort.

At least two different types of CCDs are currently available. One is a lens system with a 512 matrix, and the other is a fiberoptic system with a 1024 matrix. The latter should give higher resolution images (1).

Charged coupled device arrays are ideally suited to

S.H. Parker: Radiology Imaging Associates, Breast Diagnostic and Counseling Centre, Englewood, Colorado 80111.
R.E. Hendrick: Department of Radiology, University of Colorado Health Sciences Center, Denver, Colorado 80262.

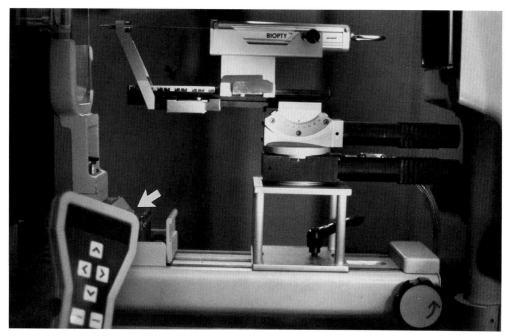

FIG. 1. "Auto-guide" automatic alignment system. The unit is motorized, so there are no manual knobs to set or scales to read. Depth is still set manually according to centimeter marks on a depth slide (*curved arrow*). A remote control device (*straight arrow*) recalls a previously digitized target and then automatically aligns the biopsy gun and needle on an appropriate trajectory. (Courtesy of Fischer Imaging Corporation, Denver, Colorado.)

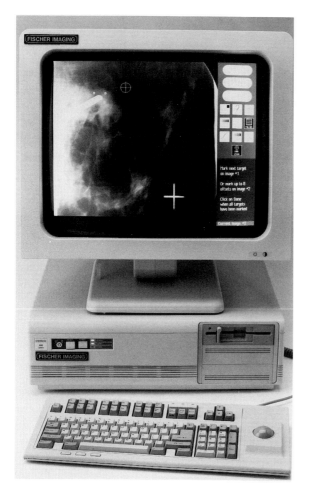

FIG. 2. Digital stereotactic mammography display. All functions performed on a digitizer are performed on the digital computer. (Courtesy of Fischer Imaging Corporation, Denver, Colorado.)

the restricted fields of view used in stereotactic localization. A 5-cm × 5-cm field of view can be optically coupled to a 1024 × 1024 CCD array, again using either lenses or fiberoptics, to give approximately 50-μm resolution at the image receptor. That resolution should permit the visualization of most small microcalcifications while improving the low-contrast resolution of solid lesions.

Another potential advantage of CCD arrays is that the image acquisition process has been decoupled from the image display process. This means that the gray scale of CCD-acquired images can be manipulated after acquisition to maximize the visibility of calcifications or lesions, potentially improving image quality. Postacquisition manipulation of image data is not possible with film. Although the CCD array, optical coupling, and computer system for image display will be added, the digitization table and the need for film and film processing will be eliminated.

There are two possible disadvantages to the CCD array digital image receptor for stereotactic procedures. One is the cost, which may be $50,000 to $100,000 higher than the cost of the screen-film system. The other is the limited field of view. With the CCD array, full-breast mammograms are not possible at this time. The user may have to switch from the screen-film image receptor used for the initial scout views of the full breast back to the CCD array during the course of a stereotactic procedure.

Other future developments include improving the sensitivity of CCD array systems by matching the spectral output of fluorescent screens to the light sensitivity of CCD arrays. Currently, conventional mammographic screens have peak spectral output in green light, whereas CCD arrays have maximum sensitivity to red light. Improved methods of coupling photon production to CCD arrays, such as making fiberoptic materials out of x-ray-sensitive fluorescent materials, are also being investigated.

ULTRASOUND

As ultrasound companies grasp the importance of breast ultrasound applications, further improvements in resolution can be expected. Although much has been written on the use of color Doppler examination to distinguish between benign and malignant breast lesions, it is our opinion, based on practical experience, that this may not prove to be as promising as initially thought. Color flow Doppler examination may, however, identify subtle lesions for biopsy more easily than does conventional gray scale imaging. Digital manipulation of images and tissue characterization techniques may further improve the ultrasound detection of breast cancer.

Large-gauge needles are relatively easy to visualize with present state-of-the-art equipment. Biopsy

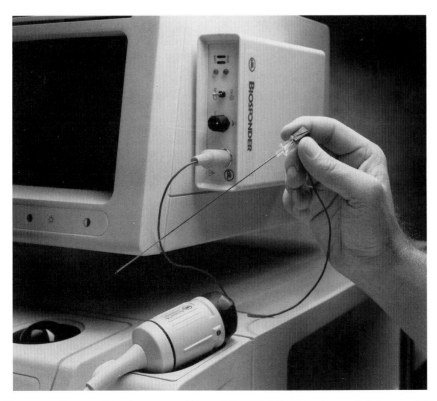

FIG. 3. Transponder needle shown configured for FNAB. (Courtesy of Advanced Technology Laboratories, Bothell, Washington.)

needles fitted with a transponder (an ultrasound crystal embedded in the tip of the biopsy needle indicating its location on the screen) may, however, make breast biopsies easier for less-experienced ultrasound operators (Fig. 3) (2).

LYMPH NODE BIOPSY

At present, surgical lymph node dissection is used to stage malignancy. The ability to diagnose lymph nodes before breast surgery could change the treatment of breast disease. Diagnosing metastatic disease in the axilla with percutaneous needle biopsy could obviate the need for surgical axillary node dissection.

Percutaneous lymph node biopsy with ultrasound guidance is easier to perform than is stereotactic lymph node biopsy (Fig. 4). (Stereotactic lymph node biopsy is discussed in Chapter 8.) If ultrasound-guided biopsy becomes accepted, ultrasonography and percutaneous biopsy of suspicious axillary lymph nodes could become part of the routine workup of patients with abnormal mammograms or breast ultrasound examinations. On rare occasions ultrasound biopsy might confirm malignancy in ultrasonographically suspicious lymph nodes in patients without visible breast lesions.

NEEDLE-BORNE TUMOR ABLATION

Local excision can be considered the definitive treatment for small (<2 cm), unifocal breast cancers. Needle-borne tumor ablation using laser therapy, ethanol injection, hyperthermia, cryosurgery, the di-rect infusion of chemotherapeutic agents, or the direct placement of radioactive seeds is a feasible alternative. These treatments, more cosmetically appealing than conventional lumpectomy, would not interfere with adjunctive therapies such as radiation therapy or chemotherapy. Multifocal, extensive, or very large cancers would still be candidates for surgical mastectomy rather than *in situ* ablation. Needle-borne tumor ablation could be guided by ultrasound, stereotactic mammography, and/or MRI.

MAGNETIC RESONANCE IMAGING

Large bore magnets and MRI-compatible needles could be used for the initial biopsy and treatment of lesions not detected on conventional breast imaging studies. Before this is feasible, however, dedicated breast MRI equipment must be developed and MRI must become more cost effective.

Early work indicates that MRI with fat suppression technique and gadolinium enhancement may be able to detect otherwise unsuspected diffuse and/or multifocal breast lesions in patients with suspicious mammograms or ultrasound examinations (3). Ruling out diffuse disease and/or multifocality before attempting needle-borne ablation is essential (see above). Thus, this may be the most significant potential application of MRI in the breast. Dependable MRI confirmation of unifocality could allow confident percutaneous ablation of unifocal cancers without the need for adjunctive therapy.

Magnetic resonance imaging may also be able to

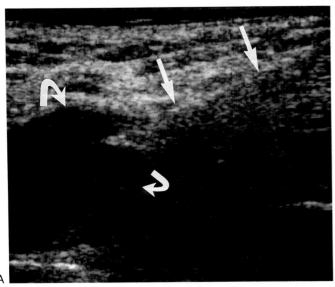
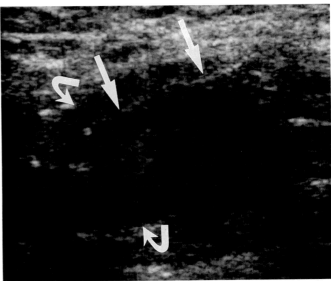

FIG. 4. Ultrasound-guided axillary lymph node biopsy. **A:** Prefire view of an axillary lymph node biopsy, with the needle (*straight arrows*) just inside the abnormal lymph node (*curved arrows*). **B:** Postfire view of an axillary lymph node biopsy, with the needle (*straight arrows*) coursing through the abnormal lymph node (*curved arrows*).

identify abnormal axillary lymph nodes or guide lymph node biopsy for presurgical staging. Site-specific coils or spectroscopy would probably be necessary for MRI to be used in this capacity.

LOWER BIOPSY THRESHOLD

In the screened population, the overall threshold for percutaneous breast biopsy could be lower than the current threshold for surgical biopsy. Lowering the biopsy threshold theoretically permits earlier diagnosis of minimally suspicious lesions. This would increase the costs associated with screening, however, and probably would not significantly affect mortality.

However, high-risk patients with strong family histories, biopsy histories of lobular carcinoma *in situ* (LCIS), atypical hyperplasia, or low-nuclear-grade ductal carcinoma *in situ* could be candidates for periodic percutaneous biopsies. Canvassing the four quadrants of the breast with core biopsy could provide minimally invasive histologic monitoring of these high-risk patients.

TURF BATTLES

Procedures involving techniques from two or more specialties, in this case image-guided needle intervention and surgical breast biopsy, unfortunately create the environment for interdisciplinary friction. The expanded role of percutaneous breast biopsy and the needle-oriented therapy that may follow closely on its heels have set the stage for just such a turf battle (Fig. 5).

The conflict between radiologists and surgeons over

image-guided, percutaneous breast biopsy can be resolved in one of two ways. As it currently stands and probably will continue, radiologists generally perform the entire procedure alone but with the support of the surgical community. Although unlikely, surgeons could assimilate the technique, virtually removing radiologists from the procedure.

In a recent survey of physicians trained at the BDCC, most radiologists reported that they perform core biopsies without surgical assistance. A small minority use an approach combining surgeons and radiologists. In many of these practices, all patients receive surgical consultation before biopsy. In others, referrals are accepted from either surgeons or primary care physicians.

Most groups performing the biopsy reported some degree of positive acceptance from surgeons in their communities, although a few experience predominantly negative reactions. Several factors influenced the degree of surgeons' acceptance or resistance. Taking a low-profile approach without directly confronting surgical colleagues seemed to be one of the biggest positive factors influencing acceptance. Entirely omitting surgeons from the "loop" naturally brought resistance from the surgical community. With the low-profile approach, the natural word-of-mouth groundswell among women themselves and among primary care referring physicians provided sufficient referrals for the procedure while reducing confrontation with surgical colleagues. In addition, in many of the communities

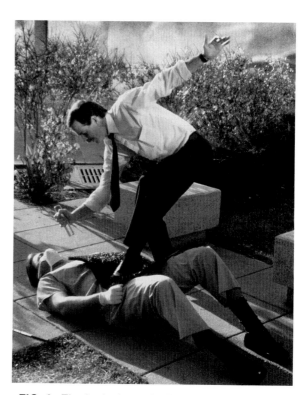

FIG. 6. The logical conclusion to the turf battle.

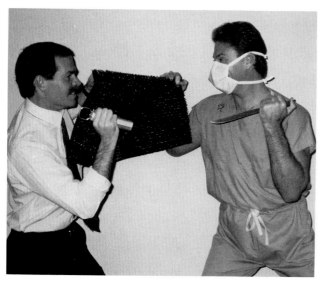

FIG. 5. Battling over the Astro turf. Will the needle or the knife win?

surgeons eventually acknowledged the technical accuracy of the biopsy and the better care it provided for their patients. Finally, acceptance occurred much more rapidly and completely in communities with very busy surgeons or in health maintenance organization (HMO)/socialized medicine settings.

Regardless of its merit a new procedure may not succeed if significant interdisciplinary friction persists. It is essential that those physicians most familiar with and adept at three-dimensional thinking, breast imaging, and image-directed needle guidance perform percutaneous biopsy of the breast. Radiologists are more likely to excel in these skills than are surgeons. Therefore, it is in the best interests of both radiologists and patients that any turf battle over percutaneous breast biopsy be resolved in favor of radiology (Fig. 6).

The trend is toward more conservative and less invasive diagnosis and treatment of breast cancer. As long as any turf battles are resolved in radiology's favor, the radiologist's interventional role in breast disease is just beginning.

REFERENCES

1. Toker E. *Design and implementation of a CCD-based digital imaging system for stereotactic mammography* [Thesis]. University of Arizona, Department of Electrical and Computer Engineering, Tucson, AZ, 1991.
2. Winsberg F, Mitty HA, Shapiro RS, Yeh HC. Use of an acoustic transponder for ultrasound visualization of biopsy needles. *Radiology* 1991;180:877.
3. Pierce WB, Harms SE, Flamig DP, Griffey RH, Evans WP, Hagans JE. Three-dimensional gadolinium-enhanced MR imaging of the breast: pulse sequence with fat suppression and magnetization transfer contrast. Work in progress. *Radiology* 1991;181:757.

Index